The Free Man's
Declaration
for
Health and Longevity

D1399965

William Campbell Douglass II, M.D.

Table of Contents

Introduction......................................1

Chapter 1: When I First Heard About This, I Was
Furious! The One Cancer Test That Could Save
Your Life...If Only You Knew About It.........5

Chapter 2: "The Number One Treatment I'd
Use for ANY Cancer Patient": Even Advanced
Stage Melanoma Patients Live Years Longer
and Better With This 'Miracle' Compound......13

Chapter 3: Rare Brazilian Compound Takes On
Free Radicals, Infections, and Even the
Most Deadly Cancer...........................23

Chapter 4: News of Astounding Natural Cancer
Killer Nearly Squashed Forever...............29

Chapter 5: When the Treatments Are Worse Than
the Disease...Breast Cancer Lies Exposed!....33

Chapter 6: Battle Cancer, Heart Disease,
Even AIDS With This Wonder Molecule..........39

Chapter 7: The All-Natural Disease-Fighter
You Already Have On Hand...Beat Cancer
for Pennies a Day!...........................49

Chapter 8: The REAL Truth About Cancer.........55

Chapter 9: The Secrets and Myths of Beating
Heart Disease................................65

Chapter 10: This Very Popular Pill is One of
the Worst Things You Can Put in Your Body 75

Chapter 11: The Great Hypertension Lie and
How to Beat It: The $30 'Cure' for High
Blood Pressure...............................79

Chapter 12: Big Fat Lies! The Truth About What REALLY Powers Your Heart......................85

Chapter 13: The Best Prescription for Heart Health: Have More Sex......................91

Chapter 14: 7 Secrets to Permanent Male Potency...93

Chapter 15: The Sexual Pitfall That Can Snare Any Man Over 50!......................111

Chapter 16: Health Miracles for Women: How to Banish Breast Cancer, Osteoporosis, Menopausal Miseries, and More...............125

Chapter 17: Health Miracles for Men: Real Prostate Solutions—Keeping Your Prostate Healthy for the Long Haul..........133

Chapter 18: One Pill in the Palm of Your Hand— And Your Prostate Protection is Set!.........143

Chapter 19: Three Reasons You Don't Need "Regular" Prostate-Cancer Screening.........153

Chapter 20: Reality Check: The Extreme Dangers of Hormone Replacement Therapy..............157

Chapter 21: 7 "Forbidden" Foods You Should Eat Every Day......................163

Chapter 22: Eat All the Fried Food You Want Without Feeling Guilty or Increasing Your Heart Attack Risk......................177

Chapter 23: Low Fat Dieters Have Higher Heart Risk......................181

Chapter 24: Do Vegetarians Live Longer Than Meat Eaters? A New Study Says, "Yes." But the Numbers Don't Add Up..............183

Chapter 25: RAW DEAL! How Fresh Milk Became a Criminal Enterprise..........................187

Chapter 26: Pork: Your One-Stop Source for Daily Vegetable Intake.......................191

Chapter 27: The Most Disgusting Thing You Could Ever Drink...............................193

Chapter 28: New Research Shows Age-Related Blindness Can Be Prevented—With Food.......197

Chapter 29: It's Not Just How Much You Eat—It's What You Eat. The REAL Secret to Diet Success: All Calories Are NOT Created Equal!...........201

Chapter 30: The Newest Scam in the Supermarket: Common Foods Are Nothing But Frauds—Protect Yourself from Phony Baloney!................. 205

Chapter 31: A Cure for Infectious Disease in a Ray of Light..............................209

Chapter 32: The Rise of the "Mystery" Disease: The Symptoms...The Cause...THE CURE.........217

Chapter 33: The Worst Condition You Don't Know You Have—And the Best Way to Make It Go Away Fast....................................223

Chapter 34: Flu Shot Madness! Why Doctors Refuse the Shot—And You Should, Too........233

Chapter 35: The "Blood Sugar Bombshell" That Could Change It All!.........................237

Chapter 36: Cut Your Diabetes Risk by 83 Percent by Choosing the Right Beverages.............265

Chapter 37: Your Guide to Beating One of Today's Leading Killers...Cure Diabetes in Three Easy Steps.....................................269

Chapter 38: The Nutrition Lesson 100 Years in the Making: Learn It Now and Stay Diabetes-Free for Good......................275

Chapter 39: Could You Be the Next Victim of Syndrome X, or—Even Worse—Syndrome H?.....279

Chapter 40: Considering Knee Surgery? Read This First! 7 Keys to Beating Osteoarthritis Without Drugs or Surgery...................283

Chapter 41: Return to the Days of Healthy Joints and Muscles..........................289

Chapter 42: The Real Miracle for Arthritis Pain...309

Chapter 43: Experience the ultimate muscle-pumper that has the fitness freaks crying,"NO FAIR!" Stay STRONG, stand TALL and feel FIT with the help of just one little secret..........311

Chapter 44: 10 More Ways to Make Life More Enjoyable by Just Saying "No" to Junk Medicine..319

Chapter 45: Big Pharma Hopes You Never Find Out About This Ayurvedic Herb That Puts Alzheimer's Drugs to Shame..................333

Chapter 46: How to Survive Your Surgery........343

Chapter 47: Have You Been a Guinea Pig for the Latest, "Greatest" Surgical Scams? Read This Before You Go Under the Knife!....347

Chapter 48: Untested...Unregulated...and Unsafe! The Real Dirt on the 'Clean' Chemical.......353

Chapter 49: The REAL Secrets to a Long Life....361

Chapter 50: Live to 100...Why Stop There?......363

Chapter 51: Can This Anti-Aging Formula Really Help You Live 20 Percent Longer? 377

Chapter 52: Junk Science Gone Wild: Are Your Supplements Driving You Blind? 383

Chapter 53: I'm Still Standing! Leading Cause of Falls in Seniors Isn't Age—It's Drugs: Your Guide to Common Pitfalls and How to Avoid Them 389

Chapter 54: Killing You Softly: Death and Dementia in the Drugs You Take Every Day! ...395

Chapter 55: How to Survive Any Disaster 401

Chapter 56: How to Survive ObamaCare: Your Guide to the Ugly Future of Medicine ...405

Wellness Directory 409

References 411

Introduction

If there's one undeniable medical fact I've learned in over 40 years of treating patients all over the world, it's this: There is no such thing as an undeniable medical fact.

As you'll see on the following pages, medicine just doesn't work that way. Human beings are simply too complex.

My point is simply this: Most of the "health advice" that appears in today's mainstream press comes from misinformed "health authorities" with little or no real-world experience.

As a result, we've been inundated with dozens of medical falsehoods that have been promoted to fact. I call it "Junk Medicine"... and I'd like to show you how to get all of these harmful ideas out of your life.

Over the years, I've practiced medicine across the globe, all starting with my stint in the U.S. Navy (where I earned my wings as a flight surgeon) then to Uganda and Russia's renowned Pasteur Institute in St. Petersburg, and many places in between, including Spain, Finland, and Turkey.

During my career, I've seen firsthand what works and what doesn't work in regard to both conventional and alternative medicine. And I've seen how government interference, political red tape, and corporate profits can interfere with important medical discoveries.

You see, unlike drug companies, pharmacists, and too many doctors today, I don't have an ulterior motive. My only aim is to help you get the information you need to keep you and your family healthy. And to help you access the best treatment when you fall ill.

The purpose of these reports is two-fold: 1) To reveal the truth about the latest Junk Medicine Myths, and 2) to hand you amazingly easy and effective ways to free yourself and your loved ones from pain and disease.

Included here are dozens of the easiest and quickest ways to filter toxic Junk Medicine out of your life. Plus, I'll show you many blacklisted medical therapies and treatments (shunned by much of the medical mainstream) that can save your life.

So much of today's most-followed health advice is unscientific hocus-pocus. It's unhealthy and unpleasant, and only the power of modern media could ever convince us to swallow it. In these reports, you'll receive doctor's orders to pitch dozens of punishing myths into the trash. You'll live longer, banish heart disease, prevent cancer, relieve your joint pain, and feel much better... practically overnight!

This is the stuff that really works. In this report, you'll find names and phone numbers, and exactly what you need to know to take advantage of these proven but often overlooked therapies.

As the editor of **The Douglass Report**, my goals are to deflate the myths and champion today's most important breakthroughs.

Welcome to **The Douglass Report**. I'm glad you've chosen to join me in discovering how easy the road to good health can be.

Sincerely,

W C. Douglass

William Campbell Douglass II, M.D.
Editor, The Douglass Report

Chapter 1:

When I First Heard About This, I Was Furious! The One Cancer Test That Could Save Your Life... If Only You Knew About It

Why are so many people dying from cancer? The sad truth: It's because the mainstream cancer industry doesn't have a way to find it early enough.

And even though early detection provides the best chance of cancer survival, the only test offering truly early detection is all but being ignored.

That's right. An extremely early detection test already exists, a test that can even accurately identify the type of cancer.

Yet when the National Institutes of Health (NIH) had the chance to support this test, they passed.

In fact, their single sentence response went something like this: "There is no such thing as a universal cancer marker, therefore this must be flawed."

The cancer test that puts all others to shame

It's not flawed. It is a real, highly successful cancer test. Not only can it detect cancer years before clinical symptoms show up, it can even tell you what kind of cancer it is.

That's right. A single blood test can accurately identify more than 20 distinct cancers, even 10 years before any signs or symptoms. And the way this test works—which we'll talk about in just a moment—virtually eliminates the risk of false positives, a terribly common occurrence with mainstream tests.

I know it sounds too good to be true—a single test that can identify nearly every kind of cancer a decade before symptoms show up. But this is the real deal.

And it could very well save your life.

How fast will cancer kill you? Hint: That's the WRONG question

You probably know someone who's been diagnosed with cancer, and chances are the prognosis was pretty short: at most a few years, more likely a few months.

That's because by the time symptoms show up, cancer is pretty advanced. And since mainstream medicine can't really detect cancer until it's big enough to see, the disease is usually pretty far along.

So the time from the oncologist's diagnosis

to complications, chemotherapy, and death is never really very long.

But the time from original onset—the very first cancer cells—to the time when mainstream medicine can correctly diagnose the cancer, the time when clinical symptoms appear, well that can take a very, very long time—up to twenty years.

And once it spreads (metastasizes)—a LATE stage in the process, then it moves much faster.

By that time, the prognosis will be bleak, something every oncologist knows.

The earlier cancer is detected, the better chances of patient survival. In fact, early detection gives you the best chance—maybe the only chance—of victory.

This single early detection test offers your best chance of survival

The cancer test I'm talking about can change everything.

- Early cancer detection, maybe decades before mainstream medicine would see it

- Accurate cancer identification, so you know where the cancer started and how best to treat it

- Accurate diagnosis, so you don't have to worry about false positives

- Easy to do, because a single simple blood test does it all

This test, the test that could help millions of people defeat cancer even before it takes a stronghold, comes from a brilliant pair of scientists, Drs. James and Dorothy Morré, a husband and wife who've devoted their lives to defeating cancer.

Weed killer inspires a young scientist to defeat cancer

Back when Dr. Morré was a teenager, he got his first job, spraying weeds at the University of Missouri with a weed killer called 2,4-D.

He was fascinated by the way the plants grew out of control, then died after he sprayed them. So, with his curious scientific nature taking hold, he tried to learn more. He came across an article about 2,4-D—and at the end it posed a challenge that that young James Morré took to heart: If it was possible to learn how 2,4-D killed plants, we could cure cancer.

He's been working on the problem ever since... and now it's solved.

You see, early in his career, Dr. Morré first discovered compounds called NOX proteins, which had been the target for the 2,4-D weed killer. He realized that these proteins were nicely regulated in normal cells...but they ran wild in cancer cells.

After many years of grueling research, he was finally able to isolate the elusive tNOX, now known as ENOX2, a form of the protein that only exists on cancer cells.

One little protein holds the key to accurately detecting cancer as soon as it starts

As you might expect, the science here is pretty complicated. But it all boils down to this:

Through their research, the Morrés realized they could detect the presence of cancer using the ENOX2 protein as a marker, because it's only produced by malignant cancer cells. Basically, if you've got ENOX2 in your blood, you have cancer cells in your body.

And then they learned something even more amazing.

Each cancer has its own distinct ENOX2. The protein has a different molecular weight depending on where the cancer originated.[1] So the test the Morrés developed not only shows whether you have cancer, it can tell you exactly where it started.

That's right, the test can accurately diagnose more than 20 different cancers, years before clinical signs show up.

It all started with lung cancer...

Back in 2006, the Morrés and their team screened blood from 421 volunteers. The group included:

- 104 lung cancer patients

- 175 smokers not diagnosed with lung cancer

- 117 randomly selected patients

- 25 healthy people

Their cancer detection test showed positive for 103 of the 104 lung cancer patients. Along with that, 12 percent of the smokers (over age 40) showed positive, though none were yet diagnosed—that ratio matches the normal incidence of lung cancer in smokers. And none of the healthy volunteers came back positive.

They saw similarly spectacular results for other types of cancers, too. Using blood samples from the Early Detection Research Network of the National Cancer Institute, the team was able to detect lung cancer, breast cancer, and ovarian cancer.

And the ongoing research has allowed them to identify more than 20 different cancers. Their test, called ONCOblot® can now detect all of these specific cancers:

Don't wait to get tested... especially if you're at risk

Chances are your doctor—even your oncologist—has never heard of ONCOblot®.

But if you're at risk for developing cancer, this test could be a lifesaver.

There are three ways to get the test, all of which require a doctor:

1. Have your doctor order a test kit

2. Contact one of the three doctors already

working with the test, and have them order the test for you:

- Dr. Leigh Erin Connealy, MD
  (949) 680-1880
  www.centerfornewmedicine.com

- Dr. Claudia Hanau, ND
  (765) 464-1545
  www.hanauholistic.com

- Dr. Kimberly Wilson, NMD
  (972) 608-0100
  innovationswellness.com

3. Send a confidential email to the ONCOblot® online physician through the website at www.oncoblotlabs.com and she will order the test kit for you.

If you use the second or third option, you will get a test kit in the mail, and take it to a lab near you to get blood drawn. The lab will complete the test kit for you and submit it for processing.

Now, this test is pricey. It costs $850 for the test alone, not including any doctor or lab fees. A lot of money, to be sure, but that's less than getting tested separately for 20 different kinds of cancer—not to mention learning about the cancer before it's too late to do anything about it.

You can find more information about ordering ONCOblot® in your Wellness Directory on page 409.

Chapter 2:

The Number One Treatment I'd Use for ANY Cancer Patient:
Even Advanced Stage Melanoma Patients Live Years Longer and Better with This 'Miracle' Compound

Dan Harding was living on borrowed time.

He had Stage IV melanoma, and his cancer had spread, now invading his lung with a large 3 centimeter tumor.

Dan was enduring standard chemotherapy on the advice of his oncologist... but it simply wasn't working. And then fate stepped in. Dan began working with another doctor, the medical director of a prominent oncology in California. And that's when everything started to change.

The medical director promptly put Dan on a robust dose of a natural cancer killer she'd been using with other cancer patients with much success.

Just six weeks later, the medical director got a call from Dan's stunned oncologist, demanding to know what she had done. Because Dan's lung tumor was completely cleared... gone.

Now the medical director routinely uses this 'miracle' compound in her melanoma patients, and many other cancer patients as well. "I can't say enough about it," she told me. "It's worked terrifically well with melanoma patients, bringing on rapid results even when they weren't responding to chemotherapy."

Malignant melanoma doesn't have to be a death sentence anymore

It causes 75 percent of skin cancer deaths.

It's lethal in about 20 percent of cases.

And unlike many other kinds of cancer, melanoma is becoming more common every year. In fact, according to the CDC, 76,250 new cases will be diagnosed in 2012... and 9,180 melanoma patients will die.

That's because unless melanoma is caught and conquered very early, this highly aggressive cancer usually spreads to other organs, often with fatal results. And conventional treatment options for advanced melanoma patients are very limited, and highly toxic.

But one natural compound can turn that all around, helping even advanced melanoma patients live better, and live longer.

High-risk melanoma patients live years longer with this natural miracle

Melanoma patients, especially those whose

disease has progressed, don't have many treatment options... and the conventional options come with terrible risks and side effects. And even with that treatment, the prognosis can be dire. But <u>this miracle called ⟨Avemar⟩ changes all that.</u>

In a groundbreaking clinical study[1], researchers showed that Avemar added nearly two extra years to the lives of high-risk skin melanoma patients. Not just weeks or months... years.

In this Phase II clinical study (with a seven year follow-up), researchers found that adding Avemar to the standard chemotherapy regimen (DTIC) for just one year gave new life to 52 high-risk Stage III malignant skin melanoma patients.

First, there were 'notably' fewer toxic side effects in the group getting Avemar along with their chemotherapy, and fewer adverse events overall. And for cancer patients suffering through treatment, that makes an enormous difference to quality of life... especially together with the precious extra time they got.

You see, the patients in the group getting Avemar lived on average nearly two years longer than the patients getting chemotherapy alone (the control group). Two years longer! Their average survival was 66.2 months, 48 percent longer than the patients in the chemotherapy-only group. Plus, the five-year survival rate (a very important measure for cancer patients) was 61.5 percent in the Avemar group, compared with only 36.7 percent in the control group. On top of that, the progression-free time (meaning that their cancer didn't get any worse) was 86 percent longer in the Avemar group—an astounding 55.8 months compared to 29.9 months for the control group.

Imagine what might have happened if they'd taken Avemar for more than just one year!

The game-changing miracle that almost didn't happen

It's not just melanoma patients whose lives can be saved. Patients with many types of cancer (breast, colon, rectal, just to name a few) have had their lives turned around by the miracle of Avemar... a true miracle, because it came very close to remaining undiscovered.

Dr. Mate Hidvegi overcame overwhelming odds to discover a safe cancer cure, unlike the poisons that were being used to attack the disease at the peril of the patients. Despite numerous obstacles and a profound lack of funding, Dr. Hidvegi did not give up. Instead, this devout doctor prayed to the Virgin Mary for guidance... and an investor. And the very next day, those prayers were answered when Dr. Hidvegi met a stranger who was willing to fund his research.

With that 'miracle' money, Dr. Hidvegi patented the process of fermenting wheat germ with baker's yeast, a discovery he called Avemar (in tribute to the Virgin Mary). Since then, more than one hundred studies confirm that Avemar really is a miracle for cancer patients... even patients who thought they had no hope.

And now, more than 20 years later, major universities have caught wind of Avemar and its stunning track record... and plans for human clinical trials are in the works. And I expect those results to mirror the positive experiences even end-stage cancer patients have had with Avemar.

"Avemar helps melanoma patients even when there's nothing else we can do"

Robert Felder went to see HSI panelist Dr. Michael Rosenbaum after his oncologist had given him the bad news: There was nothing else conventional medicine could do for him.

By then, Robert's melanoma had progressed to Stage IV and had spread substantially throughout his body. He had very little time left, and even less hope, and he felt just horrible. But despite the seemingly hopeless situation, Dr. Rosenbaum knew just the thing to help Robert.

He started Robert on AveULTRA (the newest, most powerful form of Avemar), the "number one treatment I'd use for any cancer patient." When Robert started feeling better, Dr. Rosenbaum added in his second line of defense, a special hybridized mushroom extract called ImmPower (more on that in a moment).

Finally, Robert felt like he was on the right track. He was less debilitated, and feeling better. That great feeling lasted for more than eight months—a fairly long good period for such an advanced cancer patient—before Robert took a turn for the worse.

"If only people would come to me sooner, that would really show what AveULTRA and ImmPower could do. But even with advanced cancer patients, it helps prolong life and—so important—improves their quality of life."

"They work in totally different ways, so they're even better together"

Dr. Rosenbaum thinks so much of AveULTRA, it's what he would take—without question—if he had to take one thing to treat cancer. And if he got to choose a second treatment, it would be the therapeutic mushrooms of ImmPower.

"The two work in totally different ways, so they work even better when you take them together to fight cancer," he told me.

AveULTRA works inside the cancer cells, stimulating cellular immunity, he explained. The ImmPower, on the other hand, works with your own innate immune system to help it battle the cancer. So using both as part of a cancer-fighting program can have a major impact.

Attacking cancer from all sides

Dr. Hardy had a lot to add about AveULTRA's unique mechanisms of action. For one thing, she told me, it disproportionately interferes with the cancer cell's ability to use ribose, which is needed to make RNA and DNA, a truly novel means of attack. It also increases NK (natural killer) cell activity and function. And it's nontoxic to normal healthy cells, even at extremely high doses.

And studies support Dr. Hardy's experience with AveULTRA. In fact, some studies have shown it to have cancer-fighting powers similar to those of drugs... but without the horrible, debilitating side effects. And when AveULTRA is taken along with a regimen of chemotherapy or radiation, it makes them work better, and at the same time it all but eliminates some of their worst side effects.

Now, there's a LOT of science behind how and why this compound is so very effective... So I'll just hit the highlights.

- It prevents cancer cells from repairing themselves, and that leads to cancer cell death.[2]

- It helps your NK cells recognize even disguised cancer cells, so your immune system knows exactly where to attack.[3,4]

- It can significantly reduce oxidative stress, which is often linked with the wasting syndrome suffered by advanced cancer patients[5]

- AveULTRA decreases the spread of cancer (metastasis) and substantially reduces cancer recurrence[6]

AveULTRA alone is enough to turn the tide

for even advanced cancer patients. And adding ImmPower to the mix shifts the odds even further.

ImmPower destroys cancer cells and provides powerful immune protection

Back in January 2000, there was literally only one place in America to get it. Now, with greater availability and even more science behind it, ImmPower joins AveULTRA to conquer cancer.

The key component of ImmPower is called AHCC, an extract of a unique hybridization of several kinds of medical mushrooms known for their immune-enhancing abilities. The resulting compound is so potent that dozens of rigorous scientific studies have established AHCC as one of the world's most powerful and safe immune system stimulators. Not only that, studies confirm that AHCC effectively fights many types of cancer and may even prevent recurrence of certain cancers... with no dangerous side effects. And it's been proven to have a wide range of effects on the immune system.

- Stimulating cytokine (IL-2, IL-12, TNF, and INF) production, which boosts immune function.

- Increasing NK cell activity against diseased cells as much as 300 percent.

- Increasing the number and the activity of lymphocytes, specifically increasing T-cells up to 200 percent.

- Increasing the formation of TNF, a group of proteins that help destroy cancer cells.

All that translates to more cancer-fighting power. In fact, one small clinical trial[7] showed that taking 3 grams of AHCC per day significantly decreased tumor markers (substances that detect the presence of tumors) for patients with several different types of cancer, including prostate, ovarian, multiple myeloma, and breast cancer. What's even more impressive: This study documented complete remission in six of 11 patients.

Add that to the cancer-conquering powers of AveULTRA, and cancer simply doesn't stand a chance.

AveULTRA plus ImmPower can help even advanced cancer patients survive and thrive

AveULTRA can help you fight cancer and win—and help you feel better during the fight. And perhaps most important, AveULTRA may give you more precious time, even in the most desperate circumstances.

And when you add ImmPower into your regimen, you'll be giving your own immune system the support it needs to join the fight against virtually any kind of cancer.

The manufacturer recommends using one packet of AveULTRA™ daily. Simply add the contents of the packet to four ounces of cold water or juice, mix well, and drink within 30 minutes.

(For the best tasting mixture, they recommend shaking it with ice.)

To maximize the absorption, it's best to consume AveULTRA on an empty stomach, one hour before or after eating, and one hour before or after taking any other dietary supplements or medications, including ImmPower.

For cancer patients, the research supports taking three grams of ImmPower per day to jump-start NK cell activity. It's best to take three separate doses of two capsules each: two in the morning, two at mid-day and two at night. After three weeks, the dose can be reduced to one gram per day (one capsule in the morning and one at night), to maintain the increased NK cell activity level.

For best results, take AveULTRA and ImmPower at least one hour apart. See the Wellness Directory on page 409 for ordering information.

Chapter 3:

Rare Brazilian Compound Takes On Free Radicals, Infections, and Even the Most Deadly Cancer

It's only found in the heart of Brazil, an area so small you can barely find it on a map. And in that tiny region lies the most powerful antioxidant protection you can find, a rare substance so powerful that it can stave off disease... and even many unwelcome signs of aging.

This extremely rare and unusual substance works so hard to conquer free radicals that it puts super foods like acai to shame. In fact, its antioxidant potential outstrips every food measured by the USDA.

And with all that power on your side, free radicals won't stand a chance.

Brazilian businessman stumbles across the secret to disease-free living

When Alessandro Esteves decided to trade the rat race for a peaceful life of beekeeping, he couldn't have known that his bees would hold the key to optimal health and aging. But his bees produced the most unique propolis in the world—and researchers began swarming his hives to learn its secrets.

Of course, bee propolis is a common as bees themselves—every hive creates it. But this propolis is different, and so are its distinctive healing powers. With an unmatched antioxidant profile, this propolis drew the interest of scientists around the globe. And they could only find this unusual red propolis in Alessandro's hives.

The more the researchers learned, the more excited they got. Bacteria, viruses, free radicals, cancer cells—all no match for this incredible substance.

Studies are going on even as you read this, some of them looking into just how well this rare substance fares against the most dreadful diseases.

Protecting you against the most dire diseases: Alzheimer's, heart disease, even cancer

Your body's biggest enemy may just be oxidative stress. By creating free radicals, it can bring on chronic, degenerative diseases like Alzheimer's. It can speed the aging process, even dramatically weaken your heart. And it can set you up for deadly or debilitating diseases like cancer.

And while your body has some tools to ward off oxidative stress, to really defend yourself, you need help from the outside. You need the most powerful antioxidants nature has to offer. That's the first way Brazilian red propolis protects you.

You probably know that fruits, vegetables, and spices are packed with antioxidants. And to figure out which had the most free radical fighting power, the USDA tested hundreds of foods, herbs, and spices, and calculated the ORAC (Oxygen Radical Absorption Capacity) score of each—a measure of just how well they could counteract oxidative stress and protect you against its damaging effects.

The highest scoring food was raw sumac bran, coming in at a stunning score of 312,400 (for comparison, acai scored 102,400).

But even that is no match for this unique Brazilian red bee propolis (known as FLAV™-R). That's right, based on an independent lab test, FLAV-R scored 354,000. That's a lot of muscle to help your body fight off the negative impact of oxidative stress. What's more, red propolis scored an extremely high 84.3 percent free radical scavenging ability in a standard DPPH test.

Between its unprecedented ORAC power and free radical scavenging capabilities, Brazilian red propolis has a unique ability to help your body hold off many signs of aging... and protect you against disease.

Red propolis and cancer

Some very promising research shows us that propolis also has strong cancer-fighting capabilities, against even one of the deadliest diseases known to man: pancreatic cancer.

In a groundbreaking in vitro study, researchers pitted key compounds in red propolis against extremely hard to kill PANC-1 pancreatic cancer cells[1]. Pancreatic cancer has the lowest 5-year survival rate, and is resistant to almost all known chemotherapies. In fact, pancreatic cancer thrives even when it's deprived of nutrients. But the PANC-1 cells met their match in red propolis extract, which 'displayed 100 percent cytotoxicity.' That means it was able to kill off all of the pancreatic cancer cells.

Another in vitro study[2] found that Brazilian red propolis contains cancer-killing compounds so strong they were comparably effective to common chemotherapies (including doxorubicin). Not only that, but this propolis killed off six different kinds of highly aggressive cancer cell lines, including lung carcinoma and melanoma.

What's more, in a just-published study[3], Brazilian red propolis kept human leukemia cells from growing and multiplying as well as the standard chemotherapy treatment, Gleevec.

And red propolis still brings more health-protecting potential, so your body can fight off health threats from every corner.

Antiviral, antifungal, AND antibacterial properties keep you— and the bees—in optimal health

We face a lot of threats to our health, and

so do bees. And now we have access to their virtually bullet-proof protection: propolis.

Propolis literally protects beehives from virtually all microscopic invaders. In fact, it acts as the hive's immune system, keeping the entire inner environment sterile, despite its microbe-welcoming warmth. (Bacteria, viruses, and other destructive organisms thrive in heat.)

That antimicrobial protection covers us to when we consume propolis. In fact, even rubbing it on wounds leads to quicker healing. With anti-fungal, anti-viral, and anti-bacterial powers, bee propolis can protect us against a wide variety of infections ranging from the common cold to candida (yeast) to gingivitis.

In fact, a recent in vitro study found that Brazilian propolis inhibited vulvovaginal candidiasis (the fungus responsible for vaginal yeast infections) better than some commonly prescribed antifungal medications.[4]

Try Red Bee Propolis today to give your body a fighting chance against free radicals, harmful microbes, and even cancer.

With this rare Red Bee Propolis (from Natura-Nectar, makers of EaseFemin), you'll be able to fight damaging free radicals, a broad range of infections, and maybe even cancer.

The manufacturer recommends taking one capsule daily for optimal health maintenance.

You can find ordering information for Red Bee Propolis in your Wellness Directory on page 410.

Chapter 4:

News of Astounding Natural Cancer Killer Nearly Squashed Forever

Recently, I just uncovered a remarkable story about a natural cancer killer that had been kept under lock and key for over 20 years. With this information, the future of cancer treatment and the chances of survival look more promising than ever. There's a healing tree that grows deep within the Amazon rainforest in South America that could literally change how you, your doctor, and possibly the rest of the world think about curing cancer.

Since the 1970s, the bark, leaves, roots, fruit, and fruit seeds of the Amazonian Graviola tree have been studied in numerous laboratory tests and have shown remarkable results with this deadly disease.

Several years ago, a major pharmaceutical company began extensive independent research on it. They learned that certain extracts of the tree actually seek out, attack, and destroy cancer cells. Because the natural extracts themselves could not be patented, the company labored to create a synthetic copy that showed the same promise. After more than seven years of work behind closed doors, researchers at this company realized they couldn't duplicate the tree's natural properties with a patentable substance. So they shut down the entire project. It basically came down to this—if they couldn't make huge profits, they would keep the news of this possible cure a well-guarded secret. But one researcher couldn't bear that, and decided to risk his job with the hope of saving lives.

Seven years of silence broken

This conscience-driven researcher contacted Raintree Nutrition, a natural products company dedicated to harvesting plants from the Amazon. In the course of working with Raintree on another story, they shared the exciting Graviola breakthrough with us. Since then, we've been looking closely into the research to date on Graviola. One of the first scientific references to it in the United States was by the National Cancer Institute (NCI). In 1976, the NCI showed that the leaves and stems of this tree were effective in attacking and destroying malignant cells. But these results were part of an internal NCI report and were, for some reason, never made public.[1]

Since 1976, there have been several promising cancer studies on Graviola. However, the tree's extracts have yet to be tested on cancer patients. No double-blind clinical trials exist, and clinical trials are typically the benchmark mainstream doctors and journals use to judge a treatment's value. Nevertheless, our research has uncovered that Graviola has been shown to kill cancer cells in at least 20 laboratory tests.

The most recent study, conducted at Catholic University of South Korea, revealed that two chemicals extracted from Graviola seeds showed comparable results to the chemotherapy drug Adriamycin when applied to malignant breast and colon cells in test tubes.[2]

Another study, published in the *Journal of Natural Products*, showed that Graviola is not only comparable to Adriamycin—but dramatically outperforms it in laboratory tests. Results showed that it selectively killed colon cancer cells at "10,000 times the potency of Adriamycin."[3]

Perhaps the most significant result of the studies we've researched is that Graviola selectively seeks out and kills cancer cells—leaving all healthy, normal cells untouched. Chemotherapy indiscriminately seeks and destroys all actively reproducing cells, even normal hair and stomach cells, causing such devastating side effects as hair loss and severe nausea.

Grown and harvested by indigenous people in Brazil, Graviola is available in limited supply in the United States. But now, you can be among the select few in the entire country to benefit from this powerful treatment. We encourage you to consult with your doctor before beginning any new therapy, especially when treating cancer.

Graviola has been combined with seven other

immune-boosting herbs in a product called N-Tense. As a dietary supplement, you should take six to eight capsules of N-Tense per day. Graviola and N-Tense are completely natural substances with no side effects apart from possible mild stomach upset at high dosages (in excess of 5 grams) if taken on an empty stomach.

If you've been diagnosed with cancer, you and your doctor should look into all the available treatment options. Graviola could just make all the difference in beating cancer. See the Wellness Directory on page 409 for ordering information.

Chapter 5:

When the Treatments Are Worse Than the Disease... BREAST CANCER LIES EXPOSED!

Women are being dragged to hell and back again in the name of breast cancer.

From the stress of unnecessary and harmful screenings to the poisonous drugs and disfiguring surgeries that are supposed to "cure" the disease, women are chewed up, chopped open, sucked dry, spit out and then handed a pink ribbon.

Congratulations, you're officially a "survivor." Is it any wonder that breast cancer "survivors" often have the same psychological damage as hardened combat vets?

Now, I've told you plenty over the years about the dirty secrets of the breast cancer industry, starting with the fact that the entire industry is built on a lie—the lie that breast cancer even needs treatment in the first place.

In most cases, it doesn't—but more on that in a moment, because today I want to let you in on the dirtiest secret of all: the **CONSPIRACY** to hide the toxic effects of all those unnecessary treatments—and even hide the fact that those treatments don't even work in the first place.

It starts, of course, in the mainstream scientific journals—the journals that are complicit in spreading breast cancer half-truths and outright lies. Researchers pored through 16 years of data—164 phase III clinical trials published between 1995 and 2011—and found that those studies have all the integrity of street-corner three-card Monte.

In two-thirds of those studies, researchers hid some of the worst damage of the treatment—including serious and even toxic side effects. And the more successful the trial, the more likely those side effects would be swept under the rug.

In many cases, the study authors didn't even bother to mention possible toxic side effects in the abstract (aka "the part of the study most people read"). So much for honesty and full disclosure.

A phase III trial isn't some early experiment, by the way. It's often the last stage of research before the treatment gets approved—so anything that gets left out has the chance to do serious life-ruining (or life-ENDING) damage.

And believe it or not, that's not the only little stunt researchers routinely pull.

In fact, it's not even the worst stunt they routinely pull.

When a study doesn't meet its goals, you and I would call that a failure. It's the textbook definition of the word. But cancer researchers must have a different textbook—because when a treatment fails to meet its goals, they simply move the goal. Imagine trying that in football!

Here's how it works: The failure barely gets a mention. Doesn't matter if the entire study was built around it... they'll just pretend it never happened. Instead, they'll focus on something positive that DID happen, even if it wasn't the main goal of the study in the first place.

It's a serious ethical breach, and it's not something that happens every now and again. In the 92 trials that didn't show a benefit of the treatment from the primary outcome, 58 percent simply used secondary endpoints to put a positive spin on the study.

Why do they do it? Do I even have to tell you? It's spelled:

$$$$$$$$$$$

Now, let me say up front that the study didn't find a direct link between cash and influence—but of course it didn't. Researchers don't exactly walk around wearing "FOR SALE" signs. If the influence of money were that easy to spot, the jig would've been up ages ago.

Instead of a direct cash relationship out

of the gate, it's more of an unspoken under-standing: Researchers understand that if they play ball now, the money will certainly follow, whether it's in the form of a direct grant for the next study or funding for another project at their institution.

You scratch my back, I'll scratch yours. I'd like to see someone study THAT little quid-pro-quo arrangement for a change! **_Enough_**!

This system has paid off big for both re-searchers and the drug industry—but it's been an absolute disaster for the millions of women punished by the never-ending line of bad can-cer screenings and treatments that have emerged from it.

Just look at the numbers: The rate of breast cancer detection has doubled over the past three decades, according to another new study, leading to more breast cancer treatments than ever before. But the disease's death rate has barely budged.

In the plainest of all plain talk, that means all those extra treatments aren't lives saved. They're **lives ruined**—a total of 1.3 million lives ruined through completely unnecessary cancer treatments over the past three decades, according to the new study in the **New England Journal of Medicine**.

And every year, 70,000 more women are added to that toll.

Don't let you or your loved ones be among

them. The best way to make sure you're not a victim of this scam is to avoid getting a tumor of any kind of the first place—and the easiest way to do that is to follow these four basic steps:

Skip the Mammograms: Want to turn a harmless tumor into a cold-blooded killer? Squeeze it until it bursts, and then zap it with radiation. Sounds crazy when I put it that way, right? Yet that's exactly how mammograms "work." Avoid them at all costs.

Avoid CT Scans: CT scans deliver hundreds of times the radiation of normal X-rays. And since breast tissue is more sensitive to radiation, CT scans to the chest are especially dangerous. By the way, you may hear some noise about new 3D mammograms—but they're the worst of both worlds: a mammogram AND a CT scan, all in one. No way!

Don't Work Nights: Love the nightlife? It's not loving you back, especially if that's when you work. Shift work is just about the unhealthiest lifestyle around—increasing your risk of obesity, diabetes, heart disease, and more. And in one study, even limited night shifts increased the risk of breast cancer by nearly a third.

Cut the Carbs: Tumors LOVE sugars—especially breast tumors. One study last year found that women who eat high-glycemic foods—foods that raise blood glucose, aka carbs—have a 36 percent higher risk of estrogen receptor negative (ER-negative) breast cancers. Those are the aggressive tumors that really can hurt or even kill you, so they're the ones you want to avoid most.

Finally, don't forget the most powerful tool of all: Your noggin.

Be skeptical of all the new "advances" in breast cancer screening and treatment being pushed by the mainstream, since—as I just showed you—most of them are a load of bull anyway.

This isn't just true for breast cancer... it's true of medicine in general, especially when there's Big Pharma money lurking in the background.

To find a doctor skilled in natural medicine who can help you determine the best treatment for YOU, I recommend you contact the American College for Advancement in Medicine (ACAM). You'll find them online at acam.org.

Chapter 6:

Battle Cancer, Heart Disease, Even AIDS with This Wonder Molecule

It's been called "the dollar-a-bottle miracle." It has cured drug-resistant pneumonia, eased emphysema, spared cancer patients from the miserable after-effects of chemotherapy, and rid patients of colds and flus within 24 hours. It's laughingly cheap. It's a natural substance your body already produces to fight disease (so it doesn't trigger side effects). And chances are, your doctor will never prescribe it for you.

I'm talking about hydrogen peroxide. Your own white blood cells already produce it to kill invading germs. In fact, it's your body's first and best defense against infection caused by bacteria, viruses, yeast, parasites—any foreign invader. And its method of protecting the body is both powerful and exquisitely simple. The hydrogen peroxide molecule (H_2O_2) is basically water (H_2O) with an extra oxygen atom attached. When a hydrogen peroxide molecule encounters a germ, it releases the extra oxygen atom in a process called a *respiratory burst*.

That burst oxidizes the germ, killing it.

Physicians began harnessing the curative powers of hydrogen peroxide over a century ago. In 1888, Dr. P.L. Cortelyou of Georgia successfully used peroxide to treat several nose and throat diseases. In one case, he used a peroxide nasal spray to treat a person with diphtheria—a disease that often proved fatal in that era. The person recovered in a single day.

In 1920, doctors in India were battling a particularly deadly outbreak of pneumonia. Within the Indian army, 80 percent of soldiers who contracted the disease died from it. Two doctors resorted to a highly unconventional treatment, namely injecting hydrogen peroxide directly into patients' veins. It was risky. Medical texts at the time warned that such a measure could induce a gas embolism—an extremely dangerous obstruction in a blood vessel that could cause a stroke. So the doctors only administered the treatment to patients who were considered hopeless. Out of the 26 patients given up for dead, 50 percent survived. And no one suffered a gas embolism or any other side effect.

But, as with photoluminescence, hydrogen peroxide therapy (also called oxidative therapy) stopped capturing the attention of the medical establishment once antibiotics became available in the 1940s. Isolated studies into the potential of hydrogen peroxide, however, have continued.

Clean hardened arteries and help destroy tumors

In the 1960s, doctors at the Baylor University Medical Center in Texas discovered that hydrogen peroxide could benefit both cardiac and cancer patients.

Individuals with severe arteriosclerosis (a buildup of plaque in the blood vessels) have few treatment options.

Doctors can administer chelation therapy (a process of dripping chemical agents into veins to clear blockages), but it doesn't work quickly, and it doesn't usually work on big blood vessels, such as large heart arteries and the aorta. If chelation fails, usually the only other treatment option is bypass surgery.

So the Baylor researchers set out to see if they could clear blockages with hydrogen peroxide. They dripped a solution into the leg arteries of patients with severe blockages. Later, after the patients died, the researchers did autopsies to compare the level of blockages in treated and untreated arteries. Not only had the H_2O_2 cleaned out the plaque buildup, it kept the arteries clean as well.

Autopsies showed that patients who died a year after treatment had equally clean arteries as patients who died a few weeks after treatment.

The Baylor researchers then turned to the possibilities of treating cancer with hydrogen peroxide.

They knew that oxygen plays a critical role in radiation therapy: the more oxygen a tumor contains, the more susceptible it is to being destroyed by x-rays. The researchers theorized that if they could increase the oxygen quotient of a tumor (by injecting H_2O_2 into an artery leading to it) they could increase the effectiveness of radiation treatment. Over the next six years, they treated 190 patients and saw astounding results.

One 88-year-old man with a lethal cancer on his right cheek (usually caused by chewing tobacco), was alive and cancer-free six months after treatment with H_2O_2 and radiation. With conventional treatment, his life expectancy would have been 12 to 18 months (and even less if he had opted to undergo chemotherapy).

Back in 1967, the researchers concluded that hydrogen peroxide could significantly improve the success rate of radiation therapy and the survival rate of cancer patients.

An unprecedented recovery for emphysema sufferers

Over the years, various physicians have discovered assorted uses for hydrogen peroxide. Since 1920, in fact, their discoveries have filled more than 6,100 articles in scientific journals on H_2O_2's curative powers. At one clinic, patients with high fever and influenza symptoms have seen their temperature return to normal and their symptoms disappear before an infusion of hydrogen peroxide was even completed. It has

effectively treated allergies and chronic si-
nusitis. It has eradicated the pain and helped
heal the blisters associated with shingles. It
has even helped patients with emphysema.

It's heartbreaking to see people with advanced emphysema (a progressive and fatal de-
generation of the lungs): They're painfully thin
(because they burn so much energy just trying to
breathe), their skin is the color of slate (due
to oxygen deprivation), and eventually, they
become confined to a wheelchair and permanently
connected to an oxygen mask. One particular man
was in those final, hopeless stages of emphysema when he arrived at the Douglass Center,
seeking hydrogen peroxide therapy. After four
treatments, his skin pinked up, he gained eight
pounds, and his breathing improved so much that
he discarded his wheelchair (although he kept
the oxygen mask). It was an unprecedented improvement for an emphysema patient.

I must emphasize, however, that this therapy
will not necessarily be effective in all emphysema patients. But if you ask me, it's certainly worth a try.

A new weapon in Africa's fight against AIDS

But nowhere has hydrogen peroxide therapy
proven so valuable as in Africa. In 1989, I trav-
eled to Africa and saw for myself how the AIDS
pandemic has ravaged that part of the world.
At the AIDS Clinic that colleagues and I established in equatorial Africa, I also saw the

beginning of a new medical service that could provide relief—and a future—to AIDS patients.

No one is claiming that hydrogen peroxide therapy or photoluminescence therapy can cure AIDS, or even hold off the progress of the disease. But the combination of these therapies can have roughly the same impact on AIDS as insulin has on diabetes. It doesn't cure the disease. It doesn't prevent the disease from escalating and inflicting new suffering on the patient. But it does give the patient a way to manage the disease, to keep the symptoms in check, and to resume a fairly normal life.

In Africa, we saw individuals with advanced AIDS undergo six weeks of treatment (a combination of hydrogen peroxide and photoluminescence) and recover so dramatically that they were able to go back to work.

One case was Sam, a 24-year-old veterinary assistant.

He was suffering from blurred vision, diarrhea, weakness in the joints, and severe wasting (he weighed just 85 pounds). Having already survived typhoid, high fevers, and numerous rashes, Sam was not mobile and couldn't take care of himself. But once he was put on a regimen of H_2O_2 and photoluminescence, Sam improved rapidly.

In a matter of weeks he was up and about, capable of bathing himself, and strong enough to spend 6 hours straight out of bed. It was a remarkable recovery.

There are places in this world where the only medical treatments that can be provided are those that cost no more than pennies. Hydrogen peroxide and photoluminescence are two such therapies. They constitute an opportunity to ease the suffering of millions.

Action to Take:

Hydrogen peroxide therapy has been caught in the same dilemma as photoluminescence: Politics, ignorance, and corruption have prevented this highly effective treatment from becoming widely available. To find a doctor who provides this treatment, contact ACAM. Find them online at acam.org, or call 1-800-532-3688.

Hydrogen peroxide treatments you can do in your own home

While intravenous hydrogen peroxide therapy is admittedly difficult to obtain, there are other uses of this wonderful solution that don't require wading through any medical-establishment red tape. You can use 3 percent hydrogen peroxide—the kind available in virtually every drug store and supermarket—to prevent periodontitis, erase age spots and benign moles, and clear up sinus infections, sore throats, and bronchitis.

Healthy teeth and gums at a fraction of the cost

Periodontitis isn't pretty. It involves infection and subsequent rotting of the gums around the teeth.

Obviously, no one wants this sort of thing to occur, which is why the dental hygiene business is booming. Oral care products are everywhere: You've probably seen all sorts of fancy toothpastes and mouthwashes on the shelves of your local supermarket, all of them promising (at least by implication) to keep your teeth and gums healthy.

Many brands now boast "baking soda and peroxide" as added ingredients. But why spend over three dollars on a tube of toothpaste when you can get the same—if not better—results from using the real things? The procedure couldn't be easier: Rub a mixture of 3 percent hydrogen peroxide and baking soda into your gums two or three times a day. And, on its own, 3 percent H_2O_2 is the most effective mouthwash available.

Age spots and benign moles

By nature, hydrogen peroxide is a bleaching agent. Therefore, it can be very effective for erasing any traces of brown age spots or moles from the skin.

Simply apply 3 percent H_2O_2 to the spot two or three times a day for several weeks to months.

Sinus infections, sore throats, and bronchitis

As a natural antibacterial agent, hydrogen peroxide has the ability to cure various infections. For sinus infections, use a dropper bottle to apply five drops of 3 percent H_2O_2 to each nostril twice a day (in the morning and at night). After it is snorted, the peroxide may cause a slight burning sensation. If you find this too uncomfortable, dilute the peroxide with an equal amount of water (it may be necessary to increase the dose to 10 drops if the peroxide is diluted).

For sore throats, 3 percent hydrogen peroxide used as a gargle several times a day as needed generally provides fast, effective relief.

Using hydrogen peroxide for chronic bronchitis is a bit more complicated, as it must be used with a nebulizer—a machine that will diffuse a solution into the air you breathe. (Nebulizers are available from most medical supply stores, as well as through many online sources.) For this treatment, dilute several cups of 3 percent H_2O_2 with water (a 1:1 ratio). Put the solution into the nebulizer and breathe the mist each night before bed. This procedure can be repeated in the morning as well. In addition to inhaling the nebulized H_2O_2, you should administer six drops of the same diluted solution to each nostril and snort it. Again, this may cause a slight burning sensation, which will quickly subside.

Chapter 7:

The All-Natural Disease-Fighter You Already Have on Hand... BEAT CANCER FOR PENNIES A DAY!

Eat this. Swallow that. Take this drug. Hold your nose and try to down some nasty herbal concoction with an unpronounceable name. Everywhere you turn, someone is trying to profit off your cancer fears with remedies backed by bluster and marketing, not science.

Well, it's time to cut through the bull here. The best way to beat cancer is to avoid getting the disease in the first place—and there are simple, safe, and downright CHEAP ways to make sure you never hear the "C" word from your doctor.

And it starts with something you're probably already taking—something that can cost just pennies a day: Your daily multivitamin.

One new study on 14,500 male doctors given either a multi or a placebo and tracked for 11 years finds those who took the vitamins had an 8 percent lower risk of cancer.

That's overall.

But these are men, and you know what cancer they're diagnosed with most, right? Of course you do—it's prostate cancer, the most over-diagnosed and over-treated cancer on the planet, because, in reality, it's harmless most of the time.

Turns out the multis didn't make a difference in those worry-free cancers—and once you removed all of them from the equation, the effect on everything else got much bigger.

Fifty percent bigger, to be exact—because multivitamins actually cut the risk of all cancers NOT of the prostate by a full 12 percent.

Now, you know I'm always looking for a catch in studies like this. And I found it—because this study didn't, in my opinion, use a high-quality multivitamin. In fact, I wouldn't even call it a so-so multivitamin.

The study was centered around Centrum Silver, a mass-produced multi made by Pfizer. But here's the problem with the Big Pharma approach to vitamins: They're not out to deliver a vitamin saturated with the nutrients you need most. They're out to saturate the market with a low-cost multi that people will buy based on TV commercials and flashy packaging.

Well, they delivered on that—because this stuff is cheaper than dirt (and I'll admit, the packaging is pretty good). But you get what you pay for here, because Centrum Silver contains low levels of nutrients based on laughably outdated mainstream guidelines.

For example, it contains 20 mcg of selenium, a trace mineral that's been shown to slash the risk of lung, prostate and colorectal cancers by as much as 25 percent and even cut the risk of death from cancer.

But that's in a study that used 200 mcg a day—or 10 times the amount you'll find in Centrum Silver.

It also contains 100 percent of the U.S. RDA for vitamin C, another known cancer fighter— but only at much higher levels (and to treat an existing cancer, you need even higher levels of vitamin C delivered intravenously). A high-quality multivitamin should pack in around 1,200 mg of C to be most effective. It can be challenging to find a multi with these levels, but an internet search will turn up some options like Trace Minerals' Electrolyte Stamina Power Pak.

I could go on, but the point here is that I believe the levels of major nutrients in Centrum Silver are so pathetically low that it's practically a miracle it lowered the risk of cancer by any degree at all, much less 12 percent.

So get a multi, but get one that's actually worth something. It'll cost more than Centrum Silver, but not much more—and it'll be well worth every penny.

But a multivitamin is a starting point, not an ending point—and if you REALLY want to slash your risk of cancer, you can't just take one pill and call it a day.

You'll need to do more. And you can start with my...

FOUR ALL-NATURAL CANCER FIGHTERS

Fun in the Sun: You've heard the sun causes cancer, right? Well, you've heard wrong—because the vitamin D your body makes from sunlight can actually prevent cancers, including the deadly melanomas blamed (incorrectly) on too much sun exposure. Unless you spend plenty of time outside, get between 2,000 IU and 5,000 IU of vitamin D3 each day. Some people will need even more.

Go Green: Green tea gets so much press for its cancer-fighting power that it's tempting to believe this is a triumph of marketing over science. But for once, there's plenty of substance behind the hype, because the polyphenols in green tea can prevent or fight any number of cancers. In one new study, green tea drinkers had a lower risk of cancers of the colon, stomach, and throat. In other studies, green tea has shown that it can help prevent or beat cancers of the bladder, lung, pancreas, breast, prostate, ovaries, and more. Clearly, there's something brewing here.

The 'A' Team: Speaking of melanoma, one recent study found that 1,200 mcg a day of vitamin A cut the risk of the disease by 74 percent in men and women older than 50. One of the best sources of A is the farm-fresh butter you've been told not to eat. Eat up!

Drink Up: Wine is famous for its cancer-fighting antioxidants. But if you don't like wine, feel free to drink some whiskey instead. Single-malt Scotch has even higher levels of a cancer-fighting antioxidant called ellagic acid than red wine. Even beer—especially darker brews—contains cancer-fighting nutrients. Keep the habit moderate, and you'll also slash your risk of everything from heart disease to dementia. I'll drink to that!

I've got one more for the list, but it's not something you take. It's something to **avoid**.

And it's something that's a huge part of the typical U.S. diet—which is precisely why cancer is on the rise like never before.

Sugar is practically Miracle-Gro for many types of tumors. In fact, at least a third of all tumors contain insulin receptors. That means the more sugar you eat, the faster they can grow.

The sweet stuff may even turn a harmless slow-growing tumor into a certified killer... and what makes this so much worse is that you may not even know you have a sugar-eating tumor until it's too late.

Of course, there are plenty of other ways to help slash your cancer risk. Everything from broccoli to beta-carotene can help, depending on which form of the disease you're looking to avoid.

Do your homework—and if you know you're at

risk for certain cancers, speak to a naturopathic physician about the nutrients that can
help slash that risk. I suggest one of my fellow
members of the American College for Advancement
in Medicine (ACAM).

Find them online at acam.org, or call 1-800-
532-3688.

Chapter 8:

The REAL Truth About Cancer

There's probably more Junk Medicine being circulated about cancer than about any other disease. In this chapter, I'll explain why many of these myths can be downright harmful. Plus, I'll show you a handful of inexpensive and easy things you can do to cut your cancer risk immediately.

Today's deadliest cancer myth

In the past few decades, the stigma surrounding meat has increased to epic proportions. We've been told that eating meat will kill us—one way or another. Cancer is just one of the deadly diseases that have been "linked" to meat consumption by various health "authorities." So, being the law-abiding citizen I'm sure you are, you've probably followed the government's advice to cut back on the amount of meat you eat.

But, like much of the advice given to us by the government, this is pure hogwash. Take, for example, some of the research they use to formulate their recommendations:

While decrying meat and fish as cancer caus-

ing, an Oxford University group says its research proves that olive oil will prevent cancer
of the colon. But both of the group's supposi-
tions—that olive oil is good and that meat and
fish are bad—are based on a survey so broad that
anything could be proved or disproved.

The study was based on a comparison of cancer rates, diets, and olive oil consumption in
28 countries. Sounds impressive, right? Think
again.

First, government numbers are almost always
unreliable. And due to drastic cultural differ-
ences among the countries surveyed, the uncon-
trollable variables will be massive.

Action to Take:

This is an amateurish study of no conse-
quence. Forget it. Eat all the meat you
want, with its natural fat. Rare meat is
the most nutritious, but at least stop
cooking at medium rare.

The best cancer preventive
you never heard of

The health benefits of green tea have been in
the news quite a bit lately. Two Swedish doctors from the Karolinska Institute conducted a
study that found that green tea "significantly
prevents the growth of new blood vessels in animals." This process is called angiogenesis and
is important because malignant tumors must form
new blood vessels to spread. In other words, by
drinking green tea, you can cut off the blood

supply to start-up cancer cells.

Green tea has also been proven to lower blood pressure, boost your immunity, and even prevent tooth decay.

The bottom line is that people who drink green tea every day have lower rates of heart disease and cancer... and they live longer.

Action to Take:

Drinking two glasses of tea per day is a good idea. But don't go crazy and start guzzling gallons of the stuff. There are a few circumstances, like pregnancy and wound healing in which you want angiogenesis.

But even in these situations, two to three cups a day won't hurt you.

When shopping for green tea, buy the highest grade possible. The higher the grade, the less broken the leaves. Store tea in an airtight container to prevent oxidation.

If you buy tea bags, get the ones that are individually wrapped in foil.

Give your bladder a break— and cut your cancer risk

The Junk Medicine advice pestering you to "drink at least eight glasses of water a day" is, quite literally, poisoning Americans.

Where did that 8-Glasses-A-Day advice come from, anyway? Guess what? Nobody knows!

The truth is, 1) you only need a few glasses of water a day and 2) you need to stop drinking water with so many harmful additives.

A study, conducted by researchers at the National Public Health Institute in Finland, shows that drinking normal, chlorinated drinking water—the kind that comes out of your faucet at home—causes tumors in rats. For roughly the past 100 years, chlorine has been added to just about every U.S. city's drinking water supply, because it is one way of preventing waterborne diseases, such as dysentery, cholera, and typhoid fever. Unfortunately, the risks outweigh the benefits.

Not only does the average American's drinking water contain chlorine, it also contains three other carcinogenic or artherogenic agents: fluorine, aluminum, and MX.

Action to take:

Much of the water you need actually comes from solid food. So stop drowning yourself with water... and whatever you do, stop drinking tap water.

All tap water should be filtered before you drink it, cook with it, or shower in it. Not only will filtering your water cut your cancer risks, it will also cut your risk of developing Alzheimer's disease. Tap water contains fluoride, which makes your body absorb extra aluminum.

Where does this aluminum go? Your brain. And

what metal shows up alarmingly in the brains of Alzheimer's victims? You guessed it.

Fluoridation has already been banned in Scandinavia and much of Europe... but for some reason, we still think it's a good idea here in the States.

I recommend you use an under-the-counter reverse osmosis water filter. Another option is using a water distiller.

You should also consider installing a shower filter, as some carcinogens can be absorbed through the skin or inhaled through steam.

A new cancer test that could save your life

Ask your doctor about this extremely important test, and he'll most likely say he's never heard of it. Why? Because it just hasn't been heavily promoted. But the new Anti-Malignin Antibody Screen (AMAS) is your best defense against deadly cancers.

The test couldn't be easier. Your doctor simply takes a blood sample and screens it for Anti-Malignin Antibody (AMA), an antibody whose levels become elevated in the presence of cancer cells. These serum levels tend to rise early in the course of the disease, which means you can detect the presence of cancer sometimes as much as several months—even a year—before other clinical tests find it.

Exciting? You bet. And this is not some wacky

mind-body, Zen therapy. It's been tested in studies of more than 8,000 people with amazing results.

The AMAS test can detect early cancer cells of all types. It has an accuracy rate of greater than 95 percent. With a second test, the accuracy is greater than 99 percent. (False positive and false negative rates are less than 1 percent.)

Keep in mind that the AMAS test cannot be used to diagnose cancer on its own. But it is a remarkable breakthrough for the detection of cancerous cells, which, taken in conjunction with other factors, may help doctors arrive at a more concrete diagnosis.

Action to take:

If you suspect that you have cancer or if you have other risk factors, like family history of the disease, ask your doctor to run an AMAS test. If he refuses, find a doctor who will perform the test.

You (or your doctor) can find out everything you need to know about the AMAS test by contacting Oncolab, Inc. Call (800)9CA-TEST, or go online to www.oncolabinc.com.

The fiber fraud

For some reason, in this country, we've adopted the Junk Medicine misconception that fiber is good for you and prevents colon cancer. The truth is that the effects of dietary fiber supplements and fiber-enriched foods are unknown and potentially very dangerous.

I've often compared it to iron-enriched foods: Iron supplementation is good for some anemia sufferers.

So what do food manufacturers do? Put it in food for everyone! A big mistake. All this does is increase the risk of arteriosclerosis, infection, and cancer. While the dangers of fiber aren't as clear as those associated with iron, is it really a risk you want to take? Besides, adding fiber to foods with refined carbohydrates and artery clogging vegetable fats isn't going to make these already unhealthy foods any less bad for you.

Action to take:

Avoid foods and supplements that have added fiber. Instead, get your fiber the best way possible—by eating plenty of meat!

The new magic bullet for cancer

When any new therapy comes onto the scene and is said to cure practically everything, the mainstream medical organizations become very skeptical. This is understandable: Usually, when a treatment is said to cure everything, it does exactly the opposite.

But I'm so excited about one seldom-used treatment that I've spent many years researching and practicing it, and I've even written a book on the subject.

Light therapy, or photoluminescence, is one

of the most powerful and underused treatments in the world right now. It works by stimulating the body's own immune response. Photoluminescence is a breakthrough therapy in which a portion of your blood is removed from your body, placed underneath ultraviolet light, then injected back into your body. It stimulates your immune system and reorganizes the body's defenses, which immediately begin destroying invading viral, fungal, or bacterial organisms. Essentially, photoluminescence brings the immune system back to life. It has had amazing, proven results for everything from cancer and infections to food poisoning and AIDS.

Light therapy has four parameters, or variables:

1. The amount of blood removed from the patient

2. The length of exposure to light

3. The intensity and the wavelength of the spectral energy used

4. The sensitivity of the photoactive drug used (if any)

Experienced doctors will make changes in these variables depending on your condition.

The facts are indisputable. I've seen them firsthand in my own practice. I have given several cancer patients photoluminescent treatment, and I have found it to be far superior to any other cancer treatment available. Photoluminescence has cured cases of skin cancer, breast cancer, uterine cancer, and so many others.

The amazing thing about phototherapy is that not only is it a magic bullet treatment for cancer, it is the cheapest and most effective way to treat any infection.

The problem with photoluminescence is that, while it can help many people, there's not a whole lot of money to be made with it. It doesn't require any sophisticated medical equipment, a lifetime of expensive prescription drugs, or physicians with specialized degrees.

Will photoluminescence make it into the medical mainstream? I think so, but we're probably in for a long fight against pharmaceutical companies and physicians who will see their profits shrink as this ultra-cheap process becomes more well-known. Ultraviolet therapy is a tremendous threat to the huge international drug companies, and, for that reason, I think it is being suppressed as much as possible.

But with the return of a wide range of infectious diseases, and with the increasing failures of antibiotics, I believe photoluminescence will eventually be given another shot.

Action to take:

To learn more about light therapy, see page 209.

Chapter 9:

The Secrets and Myths of Beating Heart Disease

Heart disease each year is the nation's No. 1 killer. Certain risk factors make it more likely that your heart is going to detonate. In this chapter, we'll explore the myths and real world secrets of maintaining a healthy heart.

The hidden cause of heart disease

We've been told over and over that cholesterol is the main culprit in causing the high blood pressure and obesity that lead to arteriosclerosis. But the truth is, your body needs cholesterol. It's the major building block for your sex and adrenal hormones (including DHEA, testosterone, and pregnenolone), and it helps to keep your liver and nervous system functioning properly. When you interfere with your cholesterol levels—either by restricting your diet or taking cholesterol-lowering drugs (which, by the way, have been linked to sexual dysfunction and increased risk of cancer)—the results can be fatal.

And in spite of the vision you may have of

hamburger grease and egg yolks glugging through your bloodstream, settling into the walls of your narrow, delicate arteries—fact is, it doesn't work that way. Cholesterol won't clog your arteries unless it has something to attach to, like a ridge or a rip.

Eggs and steak do NOT rip your arteries.

Cholesterol isn't the problem. There's a much greater "stealth" risk factor you should know about—the one that causes those rips in your artery walls. It's called homocysteine.

The REAL scoop on heart disease

Normally, homocysteine is used to build and maintain tissues. Your body forms homocysteine when you eat food containing an amino acid called methionine, which is present in all animal and vegetable protein. But too much in your bloodstream literally shreds your arteries from the inside out, allowing fat and cholesterol to stick... eventually leading to total blockage, followed by a heart attack or stroke.

In fact, the deadly effect of homocysteine was first discovered in 1964, when a young girl in Belfast, Northern Ireland, died at the age of 9 1/2 of a "massive coronary."

She'd suffered from a rare genetic disease that also causes seizures, mental retardation, knock-knees, and abnormally high arches. But her autopsy revealed something even more startling: She had the hardened, obstructed arteries of a 70-year-old with full-blown heart disease.

Researchers weren't sure why this had happened, but testing revealed traces of homocysteine in her urine.

They named the disease homocystinuria. Further research showed that all children who had died from homocystinuria (which occurs in about 1 in 80,000) had lesions in their blood vessels and hardened arteries.

We now know that the long-term effects of homocysteine overload in normal, healthy men are just as deadly.

The damage spreads like wildfire

Thirty years of intensive research has revealed that excess homocysteine disables a mechanism in your arterial cells called contact inhibition, which regulates the growth of the smooth muscle cells just below the inner wall of the artery.

As a result, the smooth muscle cells multiply out of control. This creates a bulge that pushes other cells apart and protrudes into the artery. This is what makes arteriosclerosis possible: The inner wall becomes uneven and rough, then the build-up of plaque begins... and the rest, as they say, is scientific.

Studies published in many prominent medical journals have linked elevated homocysteine levels with cardiac problems. An article in the June 1996 issue of *Medical Tribune News* stated the following: "High levels of homocysteine, a substance involved in protein production, are associated with artery thickening, a precursor to both stroke and heart disease."

A team of cardiologists in Norway conducted a study in which they followed 587 heart patients for five years. The results, published in *The New England Journal of Medicine*, showed that 24 percent of the patients with high levels of homocysteine in their blood were dead within five years. The five-year mortality rate among the patients with normal homocysteine levels was only 3 percent.

A 1992 Harvard study of 15,000 physicians showed that those physicians with the highest 5 percent of homocysteine readings had a three-fold-plus increase in heart attack risk (JAMA, vol. 268, pp. 877-81).

Homocysteine also interferes with your blood vessels' natural ability to relax and makes your blood stickier.

The good news is that there's a simple secret to controlling homocysteine overload: Your body requires a steady supply of three particular "helper nutrients" to process, convert, and excrete excess homocysteine.

The three Bs for better vascular health

Vitamins B6 and B12 and folic acid (which is also a B vitamin) are the keys to maintaining normal homocysteine levels. These three nutrients play a crucial role in converting the potential villain homocysteine into cystathione and methionine, which are harmless.

Folic acid is the most important of these B vitamins in attacking and neutralizing homo- cysteine. There are studies reported in peer- reviewed international medical and research journals that demonstrate the benefits of folic acid to help keep homocysteine levels healthy.

Action to take:

The bottom line is that you need all three nutrients to keep your homocysteine levels healthy. Folic acid and vitamins B6 and B12 are readily available in citrus fruits and in fresh leafy green vegetables like spinach. But because I believe our foods are so over-processed and our soil is seri- ously depleted of nutrients, it's important to fortify dietary sources with nutrition- al supplements, including 800 mcg of folic acid along with vitamins B6 and B12 per day. Folic acid and B-vitamins are available in most vitamin and health-food stores.

Blocked arteries don't cause fatal heart attacks

Here's a deep, dark secret that bypass sur- geons hate to admit: When autopsies are per- formed on dead heart attack victims, they often find no blocked arteries at all!

Isn't that curious? Everyone tells you that fatal heart attacks are always caused by hard- ened arteries. But postmortems show us it's just not so.

Here's another fact they're unlikely to tell you. The respected journal, *Circulation*, reported that most patients with blocked arteries actually grow their own bypasses.

How? When your body discovers a blocked artery, it sends out a message to your arteries, telling them to grow a network of smaller, collateral vessels. In most patients, these new vessels compensate perfectly well for the clogged ones.

A new heart care revolution is gaining momentum

Medical science has rediscovered a remarkable nutrient that may do wonders for the heart, Terminalia arjuna.

This one herbal extract can help support healthy circulation, blood pressure and cholesterol levels.

Chances are you haven't heard of arjuna yet. But I can assure you it won't be long before some news rag claims discovery of the "newest" breakthrough in heart health history. In actuality, arjuna is an Indian medicinal herb that's been traditionally used as a supporter of strong heart function for more than 2,500 years.

How to expand your arteries almost instantly after every meal

Vitamins, believe it or not, can have an immediate and powerful effect on your blood vessels. They negate the effects of high-fat foods: Cardiologists have found that taking high doses of vitamins C and E before a high-fat meal will help your blood vessels dilate properly.

In a study at the University of Maryland, subjects were divided into two groups. One group was given vitamins, the other wasn't. Both groups were then fed high-fat meals. Researchers found that the blood vessels in subjects who had taken vitamins remained dilated well after the meal, while those who did not take vitamins saw their dilation drop by as much as 33 percent.

Author of the study, Dr. Mary Corretti said: "Our study raises the interesting possibility that we may be able to influence minute-by-minute changes that occur in blood vessels that lead to the heart and blood vessel disease."

Action to take:

Take 500 mg of vitamin C and 400 IU of vitamin E each night at bedtime.

Clean out diseased arteries permanently, without surgery, dieting, or drugs

Ask your doctor about this therapy, and he'll probably say it's "quackery." You can call it whatever you want, I only know that it works. I've personally treated many patients with it and have seen their positive results.

I'm talking about chelation therapy.

The theory behind chelation therapy is that

it causes certain chemicals in the body to bind with calcium and other toxic metals and then flushes them out of your system. Once the calcium is out, plaque (which is laden with calcium) will slowly dissolve—essentially cleaning out your arteries and improving the blood flow.

This is, of course, a very simplified explanation of how chelation therapy works. And, in fact, the more we learn about it, the more questions we have.

The main agent used in chelation therapy is called ethylenediaminetetraacetic acid, better known as EDTA.

It's commonly used as a food stabilizer, and you'll most likely find it listed on the label of the mayonnaise jar in your refrigerator.

One of the most amazing chelation stories I've personally been involved with is that of a friend of mine.

Nineteen years ago, his doctors told him his arteries were so clogged that his death was imminent. He was a lawyer from Wheeling, West Virginia and, like most smart people, he went looking for a second opinion.

In the years since, he has had more than 400 chelation treatments. Today, he feels great.

Before beginning chelation therapy, your doctor should check for kidney malfunction, heart failure, and other problems that would indicate you need to be careful about your treatment.

After that, the chelation treatments themselves are actually very simple. It's simply a matter of sitting still and hooking up to an IV. Usually, doctors will have you sit in a reclined position for several hours with an intravenous drip.

Actions to take:

Watch how much iron you get in your diet. If you can find a doctor who understands the importance of iron, get him to check your ferritin level (iron status).

Contact the American College for the Advancement of Medicine at (800) 532-3688 for a referral to a doctor near you who can help you with chelation therapy.

If you decide to undergo chelation therapy, I recommend you commit to 30 treatments. And don't expect a miracle overnight. Remember, the plaque in your arteries wasn't built in a day.

Chapter 10:

This Very Popular Pill is One of the Worst Things You Can Put in Your Body

From here on out, any medical professional who recommends statin drugs to healthy patients is either delusional or in denial (or borderline criminal!). Either way, it's time to get over it.

I'm not talking about the known risk of statins raising blood sugar and promoting type 2 diabetes (although that alone is all the reason you need to avoid statins).

And I'm also not talking about the known risk of statins causing cognitive problems (usually referred to as "brain fog" to make it sound more cute than dangerous).

This time I'm returning to familiar territory: muscle pain.

But "pain" hardly begins to describe what's going on here. Some of these cases of pain lead to fatalities. And if you're like me, you'll find it hard to believe who is at greatest risk of experiencing statin-related muscle pain and all the complications that can go with it.

We've known for many years that statin use increases risk of muscle pain and fatigue.

Then, a few years ago, studies revealed that pain and fatigue are actually symptoms of something much more serious: muscle damage. As the alarming warning on the Lipitor website puts it, this damage "can lead to kidney problems including kidney failure."

And just to be clear, kidney failure is not a condition you come back from—it's the absolute end of the line.

But now the issue of muscle damage has taken another leap forward with this astonishing new warning: People who exercise are the ones who are most likely to experience statin-related muscle pain. And the more you exercise, the greater the pain, and the greater the damage.

According to a *New York Times* report, about 10 percent of statin users experience muscle ache, pain, or fatigue. But among people who exercise regularly, that percentage rises to 25 percent. And the rate is an astonishing 75 percent or more among competitive athletes.

Of course, the irony here is subtle as a sledgehammer, because regular exercise is one of the healthiest and most effective means of controlling cholesterol levels. Most doctors who write a statin prescription will advise you to start getting daily exercise. But many patients who begin taking the pills will soon be feeling fatigued and unmotivated—unlikely to get a daily exercise regimen off the ground. And then, those who push themselves to exercise despite the fatigue, may actually cause greater harm to their muscles than if they just sat on the couch and watched TV.

This insidious pattern was recently confirmed in a French study where researchers compared muscle biopsies from mice given statins vs. mice who didn't receive the drug.

In mice that weren't exercised, oxidative stress (which is a measure of potential cell damage) was 60 percent higher among the animals that received a statin compared to those who didn't.

In mice that were exercised on treadmills, muscle oxidative stress was more than 225 percent higher among the animals that received statins. In addition, the biopsies showed evidence of dysfunction in cell mitochondria, the mechanisms that generate a cell's power.

One cardiologist told the Times that it appears that statins not only increase muscle damage during exercise, but afterwards as well. And what's worse, the drug may actually interfere with the body's ability to repair damaged muscles.

As with the increased risk of type 2 diabetes, and increased risk of cognitive problems, the worst part of this muscle damage issue is the fact that most people who use statins don't need them at all.

Evidence shows that a small percentage of statin users who have known cardiovascular problems will benefit from a slightly reduced risk of fatal heart attack. But for those who have high cholesterol and no other cardiovascular problems, statin benefits are virtually nonexistent.

It's time for doctors everywhere to let go of their statin dependency and put it behind them. It's done.

Chapter 11:

The Great Hypertension Lie and How to Beat It: The $30 'Cure' for High Blood Pressure

High blood pressure isn't a disease. It's a phony-baloney excuse to drug as many people as they possibly can, and the proof is in the pudding.

Or in this case, the proof is in the guidelines.

They're changed more often than American Idol judges, but they haven't resulted in healthier people—only more people who take blood pressure meds.

And that's because the guidelines for hypertension—*the very guidelines your own doctor relies on to make treatment decisions every single day*—aren't carefully crafted by teams of independent researchers.

They're schemed up by "experts" who pocket big money from Big Pharma—and since they don't want their ride on the gravy train to end, they keep changing the guidelines to please their benefactors.

So down, down, down the BP targets go—and eventually, they trickle down to you.

One day, your BP is fine. The next, it's exactly the same—but now it's dangerously high, thanks to new guidelines, and your doc is handing you a prescription for a pricey new drug. (It's never the cheap old stuff, is it?)

It's easy to think you just can't win. But you can—and all you need is a little information. Information that you can get... but your doctor can't.

And it starts with understanding why your blood pressure changes in the first place.

For most people, blood pressure levels aren't constant. They're changing all the time... rising... falling... rising... falling... more of a roller coaster ride than a flat line, and the high points on that ride are almost always during trips to the doctor's office.

It's the stress of being in the clinic.

Maybe it's all the poking and prodding. Maybe it's the needles and blood tests. Maybe you're always expecting bad news. Maybe it's the surly receptionist, the co-pay, the paperwork, the guy hacking up part of his lung in the waiting room, the hunt for a parking spot, or some combination of all the above.

Whatever the reason, BP that shoots up in the doctor's office is so common that it has its own medical name:

White Coat Syndrome

Sounds ominous, right?

It's not. All that means is blood pressure that's high in the presence of a white coat— aka your doctor—but perfectly normal most of the rest of the time.

The only problem is, no one is checking your BP levels most of the rest of the time.

But you can change that easily enough. Take your readings at home, hand them over to your doc and—just like that—your hypertension could be "cured."

Don't think it's that simple? Trust me, it IS that simple—and the science backs me up here.

One study just last year tracked 444 patients for 18 months, with BP levels measured throughout the study in three different settings—at home, at a doctor's office, and in a research lab.

Only a third of the patients in the study had consistent numbers. The rest were riding that roller coaster, showing all the ups and downs I just told you about—with many of the biggest ups coming in the doctor's office.

But here's the most important piece of information from the study: The average patient had numbers that would be considered hypertension whenever the doctor took the reading.

Their systolic reading—that's the top number—hit 145, or well past the 140 that supposedly marks the start of the condition, at least according to guidelines.

Outside the clinic, however, that number plunged to an average of 130, or just high enough that you might get a frown and a lecture from your doctor (feel free to ignore it)... but low enough that even the strictest guideline-following hack won't try to drug you (and run the other way if he does).

Remember, these weren't the atypical patients—these were the averages, and other studies have reached very similar conclusions.

Clearly, you need to take matters into your own hands and take readings outside of the doctor's office. But don't waste your time using the free machines at the local pharmacy or senior center.

For around $30, you can get a reliable automated device you can use at home. If you want to spend more, you can get devices that'll do everything but make your coffee—devices that can talk to your computer, your iPhone, and your iPad, and some that can even send your readings right to your doctor's office.

Take your measurements, and then tell your doc to read 'em and weep.

But what if it doesn't work?

OK, so while most people will find their BP

levels are lower at home, not everyone will. And if you still have teenagers at home, it might even go up.

If that's your story, it's still not time to panic.

Like I said earlier, the guidelines themselves are badly flawed. Right now, anything over 140/90 is considered hypertension, and there's a push to lower it to 120/80. But the science here is clear: You could go higher than 140/90—much higher—**and face no increased risk at all**.

A recent Cochrane review looked at data on some 9,000 people who took part in drug trials in the United States, Britain and Australia. They all had "hypertension," with systolic readings of between 140 and 159 and diastolic readings of between 90 and 99.

The vast majority of "hypertension" patients fall within this range, and most of them get drugs to bring those levels down.

But if that range was such a danger zone, surely people who aren't drugged would be dropping dead of heart attacks all over the place, right?

WRONG!

According to the study, patients who were given placebos and patients who were given no treatment all had the exact same outcomes as the ones who were drugged.

Same risk of heart disease... same risk of heart attack... same risk of stroke... and the same risk of death.

The only difference came in side effects—patients on meds got oodles of them, of course, and for nearly 10 percent the side effects were so bad they had to stop taking the drugs.

Looks to me like they were better off without them anyway.

Of course, there comes a point when BP can get too high—and BP that suddenly shoots up and stays up in the stratosphere can be a warning that something in your body needs attention.

In those cases, taking a med to lower your BP is like turning up the car radio so you don't hear the police siren behind you. It might make the symptom disappear... but it won't change the fact that you're in trouble.

So forget drugs and work with an experienced naturopathic physician who can figure out what caused your blood pressure levels to spike. Once he finds that cause, he can help you to correct it.

Isn't that how medicine is supposed to work?

I recommend visiting one of the enlightened doctors of the American College for Advancement in Medicine. To find one near you, call 1-800-532-3688 or visit them online at ACAM.org.

Chapter 12:

BIG FAT LIES!
The Truth About What REALLY Powers Your Heart

You've been told for years that saturated fats are unhealthy... lectured like a child about the so-called dangers of red meat... and even **threatened** with disease and death if you ignore government advice and eat meats and dairy anyway.

Saturated fats have been so vilified that I'm surprised the USDA hasn't launched drone strikes on cows and pigs (and yes—believe it or not, the USDA has drones).

Well, next time you hear the lectures—next time you hear the LIES—tell 'em to stick a fork in it. Then, stick a fork into your steak and enjoy every healthy bite—because new research confirms that saturated fats are critical to your heart.

In fact, the study proves that cutting back on these fats isn't just unhealthy...

It's downright suicidal!

Researchers split 458 middle-aged men who

had recently suffered a heart attack or angina into two groups.

The first group was told to keep eating saturated fats. Your own doc (not to mention the government know-it-alls) would probably call that crazy—but if you want to see something really insane, take a look at the second group.

They were told to cut saturated fats to less than 10 percent of their daily calories. Then, they were ordered to replace those healthy animal fats with polyunsaturated fats from plant and seed oils.

For example, they had to replace honest-to-goodness butter with a safflower oil-based margarine, bringing their polyunsaturated fat intake up to a minimum of 15 percent of their daily calories. These changes also caused their levels of essential omega-3 fatty acids to plunge, while raising their levels of omega-6.

Do I even need to tell you what happened next?

The men who made the so-called "healthy" switch saw their cholesterol levels plunge by 13 percent. They must've been thrilled. Their doctors must've been ecstatic.

They were probably ready to celebrate, and then...

They started dropping like flies!

They died off at **DOUBLE** the rate of the heart patients who were allowed to keep eating saturated animal fats. They had a higher risk of death from all causes, and more specifically a higher risk of death from heart disease and other heart problems, according to the study in **BMJ**.

Funny thing about this study, by the way: It was conducted between 1966 and 1973—at the dawn of the low-fat "revolution," when governments and Big Ag converted everyone to the false gospel of grains, soy, canola, and safflower.

But the study was only published this year.

What happened? Supposedly, the data was "missing" and only recently rediscovered.

Maybe that's even true... but I suspect someone saw the results and thought the study might be a career-ender, since it was so out of tune with the emerging mainstream message.

And we've been killing ourselves with that message ever since.

Clearly, it's time to change that message and get back to basics—but it's not as easy as swapping margarine for butter anymore, because something else has happened over the past few decades.

We started treating cows as badly as we treat ourselves.

Once upon a time, cows were set loose and allowed to munch on grass all day—a lifestyle perfect for producing milk and meat with high levels of critical omega-3 fatty acids and low levels of omega-6 fatty acids.

Today, the animals on factory farms eat the same

junky diet of plants, grains, and seed oils that has wrecked human health. This has literally re-engineered cows, causing them to produce meat and milk with dramatically higher levels of omega-6 fatty acids and almost none of the essential omega-3s.

So while ANY butter is better than margarine and ANY meat is better than tofu, the best way to get the essential nutrients and healthy animal fats you need is by getting them from grass-fed cows instead of the animals raised on factory farms.

Don't shy away from the fatty cuts, and enjoy full-fat RAW dairy instead of the pale run-off that passes for milk in supermarkets.

If you want to nibble on a plant or two along the way, be my guest—but do it because you want to, not because you have to. And if you really want to turbo-charge your heart protection plan, follow my...

FOUR STEPS TO ULTIMATE HEART HEALTH

Don't Fear the Shaker: The saltshaker, that is—because the idea that salt causes heart disease is medical myth, not science.

In fact, the science is crystal clear on this. Dozens of studies have proven that LOW-salt diets are dangerous and even deadly—and one recent study in the *Journal of the American Medical Association* finds that people with the lowest sodium intake are actually <u>five times more likely to die</u> of cardiovascular disease than those with the highest.

Low sodium can also lead to brittle and broken bones, among other health problems—and let's not forget the biggest risk of all: bland and tasteless food.

Yes, it's possible to get too much sodium if you eat processed foods all day—but if that's your diet, you've got much bigger problems than salt intake anyway. Stick to real fresh foods instead, and you can shake as much salt onto it as your taste buds crave.

Get Married: Your spouse might drive you nuts at times, but married people have healthier hearts and are more likely to survive heart problems when they do strike. One recent study finds single men are up to 66 percent more likely to have a heart attack and up to 168 percent more likely to die within a month of having one.

Ladies, your numbers are pretty much the same.

I'm sure part of the reason is that happiness is good for your heart. But the rest of it is what I call the "nag factor."

That's the ability of a spouse to nag you to see a doctor when you don't want to... or to go to the hospital when you think you're fine... or to call the ambulance even as you insist that it's not chest pain, just "something you ate."

Being married will also help you out with this next tip...

Have More Sex: They say exercise is good for the heart, but that's bunk. There's a reason gyms were among the first places to install AEDs (automated external defibrillators), and it's because all that exercise brings hearts right to the brink of the breaking point.

So forget working out in the gym. The best way to stay fit is through natural movement. And the most natural movements of all are the ones that take place between the sheets.

Studies have shown that sexually active adults have stronger, healthier hearts. In fact, men who "do it" at least twice a week have half the risk of heart disease of men who do it once a month or less.

And if you've already had a heart attack, don't worry. Not only will sex NOT cause another one, but studies have shown it can actually help prevent that second attack.

The general rule of thumb for heart attack patients is that once you're healthy enough to climb a couple of flights of stairs, you're healthy enough to climb back into action in your bed.

Raise Your Glass: Moderate drinkers have healthier hearts, period.

One study out of Spain found that men who drink daily are 50 percent less likely to develop heart disease than men who don't. And if you've already had a heart attack, don't stop.

Moderate drinking can cut the risk of a second heart attack in half, slash your risk of death from heart disease by 42 percent and even help reduce the risk of death from all causes by 14 percent.

Salud!

Chapter 13:

The Best Prescription for Heart Health: Have More Sex

If you want to gobble down aspirin because of some imaginary heart benefit, be my guest. But if you really want to aid your ticker, spend more time in bed instead (and I don't mean sleeping!).

Go ahead... give that mattress a workout—because a new study shows why sex is the only form of steady exercise I endorse. Men who do the deed at least twice a week have half the risk of heart disease compared to those who do it once a month or less.

And if you think the men who do it more often have a lower risk because they're healthier to begin with, then you're as innocent as a virgin. The researchers adjusted for risk factors like age, weight, and blood pressure... and found that having plenty of sex still made all the difference in the world.

I can't say I'm surprised. It doesn't take a genius with a research grant to figure out that sex is more than just a sweaty diversion. It's mankind's oldest wonder drug, and men and women alike can share the benefits.

Steady sex can reduce stress, fight pain, and energize the immune system, making the body more capable of fighting cold and flu. Forget flu shots, the best injection takes place in the bedroom!

Side effects: happiness and physical exhaustion.

So stop reading and get busy—your life depends on it.

Chapter 14:

7 Secrets to Permanent Male Potency

No one wants to admit it, but for many people a lagging libido is a major problem. Face it, we're not as young as we used to be... but that doesn't mean we're no longer entitled to satisfying sex lives.

There are a number of steps you can take to regain the level of intimacy you had when you and your spouse were newlyweds.

What kills your potency and libido?

Homocysteine. Over 30 years of research has proven that high amounts of homocysteine produce ridges, tears, and protrusions that allow cholesterol to do its damage.

Plaque builds up on these ridges and leads to atherosclerosis, or clogged arteries, which leads to insufficient blood flow to all organs of the body, including the genitals. The result could be a weak or nonexistent erection and lack of vaginal engorgement necessary for stimulation.

Thankfully, improving your vascular health

may be easier than you think. While doctors like to paint pictures of steaks, hamburgers, and eggs clogging your arteries, this is not the way it works. In fact, your body needs cholesterol for good sexual functioning. It's the major building block for your sex and adrenal hormones.

So you can eat your steak, as long as you follow what I call the "three Bs to better vascular health." These are vitamins B6, B12, and folic acid (which is also a B vitamin).

These three nutrients play a crucial role in converting the potential villain homocysteine into the harmless, naturally occurring amino acids cystathione and methionine.

Prescription and over-the-counter drugs. If you take prescription acid-blockers or antidepressants, you could be making yourself impotent and lessening your libido. Luckily, there are natural alternatives for these medications.

One such substance is an extract of rice-bran oil called gamma oryzanol. Listed in the Merck index as an anti-ulcerative agent, Japanese researchers have found that it can greatly accelerate healing of a range of gastrointestinal ailments. In a Japanese study conducted at 375 hospitals patients given 300-600 mg of gamma oryzanol experienced better healing of their ulcers and a faster recovery than patients on conventional medication. You'll likely find gamma oryzanol supplements at your local health-food retailer.

In one open trial, Ginkgo had a positive effect not only on erections but also on libido and orgasm--so women may find it to be a major help as well.

The quantities used in the study ranged from 60 mg per day to 120 mg twice a day. The best way to supplement with the herb is to start with a lower dosage and work your way up if the results aren't significant. Check with your doctor before starting on Ginkgo, as there are some side effects to Ginkgo usage, such as headaches and gastrointestinal problems. You can buy Ginkgo at most health-food, discount, and grocery stores.

Testosterone loss. As men get older, the amount of testosterone in your blood drops gradually—about one percent per year after age 40. As a result, your performance can start to slide. The machinery still operates, but with less energy. There are three immediate signs of low testosterone levels: 1) the increase of fat around your middle, 2) loss of muscle, and 3) loss of bone density.

As men age, their testosterone levels decrease, their testicles shrink and their prostates grow, swelling with hard connective tissue that complicates urination and ejaculation.

While testosterone is thought of as a male hormone, women's bodies also contain it, and its presence is essential for overall good health, as well as for sexual function. Loss of testosterone can result in lagging libidos for both sexes.

But you don't have to live with it.

Increase testosterone naturally

Human growth hormone (HGH), which causes your body's glands to produce more of the hormones (including testosterone) that reverse the aging process, is riding the current wave of prescription drugs for increasing muscle mass and turning back the clock. But instead of spending five figures for a year's worth of shots, you can get HGH for free. Strength training increases HGH production more than any other type of exercise.

Higher rates of HGH flooding your body increase the rate of cell and tissue repair. As your muscles break down with strength training, HGH repairs and rebuilds the tissues and cells—via the process of building muscles and fighting the degenerative effects of aging.

While HGH is going up and flipping the calendar in reverse, your testosterone level is also rising to meet all the demands of your more youthful body.

Consider traditional supporters

Maca. This South American herb has a long history of use for promoting healthy levels of libido. One early study conducted with mice show positive results for sexual function using maca extract.

Korean red ginseng. Researchers have shown

that long-term use of this herb can support a man's capacity to have an erection. You can buy Korean red ginseng at most health-food stores.

Vitamin E. This contributes to the health and longevity of your sex drive. It's found in cod liver oil, nuts, and fresh fish like salmon.

DHEA. Less tested as a way to prevent testosterone deficiency, but not lacking in endorsements, is dehydroepiandrosterone (DHEA), which is your body's most plentiful hormone. Like testosterone, it floods your body when you're young and dimishes as you grow older.

DHEA fuels the production of sex hormones—particularly testosterone—and thus is a less powerful alternative to the testosterone patch. Believers swear that restoring youthful DHEA levels improves their memory, mood, energy, and sex drive—even building lean, healthy body mass.

Researchers at the University of Mississippi Medical Center demonstrated that doses of DHEA regulated growth of prostate tumors in mice while boosting their sex drives!

DHEA formulations are now available over the counter in most health-food stores. However, you should work with your physician whenever supplementing with hormones.

Muira puama. This South American herb is also known as "potency wood." Originally used by traditional tribal healers, muira puama has now joined the growing list of useful rainforest legends.

Catuaba. The bark of the catuaba tree has been used as a sexual stimulant for many years by the Tupi Indians in Brazil. According to Michael van Straten, noted British herbalist and naturopath, catuaba is beneficial to both men and women as a sexual stimulant.

Ashwaganda. This herb is known as an adaptogen, which means that it goes to where your body

---

Checking your testosterone levels: For men

Researchers at the St. Louis University School of Medicine developed a simple questionnaire that will give you a rough idea of whether or not your testosterone levels are flagging.

- ❏ Have you noticed a decrease in your sex drive?
- ❏ Are you experiencing weaker erections?
- ❏ Are your energy levels lower than they used to be?
- ❏ Are you experiencing a decrease in strength and endurance?
- ❏ Have you been getting shorter?
- ❏ Are you losing some of your "enjoyment of life?"
- ❏ Are you sad or grumpy?
- ❏ Have you noticed deterioration in your ability to play sports?
- ❏ Do you fall asleep after dinner?
- ❏ Is your work performance falling off?

If you answered "yes" to question 1 or 2 or "yes" to four or more questions overall, you may be a candidate for testosterone replacement therapy, according to the St. Louis medical researchers. If most of your answers were "no," your testosterone level is probably right up there with that of the latest teenage rock star. You should be rollerblading on the boardwalk instead of reading this.

needs help most and offers its support. Ashwaganda is also known for its energy-stimulating and stress-reducing properties, both of which can help make the time you spend in bed more enjoyable.

ASD. If you're after faster results, try androstenedione (ASD). ASD is a metabolite of DHEA made in yourbody by the gonads and the adrenal glands. The conversion of ASD to testosterone is the final step in the synthesis of sex hormones in the gonads.

ASD supplements were secretly developed by East German scientists to boost the performance of their athletes. Declassified documents show that the team of biologists, physiologists, and physicians in charge of the performance of East German Olympic athletes experimented extensively with ASD.

They found that ASD caused testosterone levels and athletic performance to skyrocket almost immediately.

If you have determined that your testosterone level is low, you may want to try ASD. Take between 100 to 200 mg per day in divided doses. Try a 25 mg capsule with each meal, with an additional capsule before exercise. Researchers recommend that you should not exceed 200 mg a day, taken three to five times a week. How you feel and perform is your best guide.

But be sure to work with your doctor to monitor your response and adjust your dosage as needed.

Gotu kola. This herb has strong antioxidant properties that help protect genital tissues from "wear and tear." Gotu kola has a long history in various parts of the world as an energy and libido booster.

Ginkgo, damiana, and **Avena sativa** are also well known as traditional herbal sexual stimulants. They have been used to incite sex drive, increase potency, promote hormonal balance, increase energy and endurance, and promote proper circulation. You can buy these herbs as either supplements or extracts at your local health-food store.

Mineral helps enhance performance

If your testosterone levels have dropped, you might want to consider supplementing with zinc. Zinc is particularly important, not only because it helps promote healing and growth, but also because it helps promote healthy levels of testosterone.

In a cross sectional study conducted at Western Washington University with 40 men ages 20 to 80, low testosterone levels were found to be positively correlated with low serum zinc levels (*Nutrition* 1996;12(5): 344-8). After the older men in the test group were given zinc supplements for six months, their testosterone levels increased!

Another mineral you may want to consider taking along with zinc is magnesium, which helps maintain healthy muscles.

The 3 secrets to MAXIMIZE your manhood

Don't let them tell you you're too old for massive muscle mass, the best sex of your life, and a power stream that would make a race horse jealous! Here's how to get all three:

#1: Experience the ultimate muscle-pumper that has the fitness freaks crying "NO FAIR"!

I've been singing the praises of creatine, an amino acid, for years. You might think only body-builders need creatine (or "body preeners", as I call them). But in my opinion, creatine is of little or no value to body builders—but it is of tremendous value to the elderly.

Creatine supplementation, with moderate weight lifting, adds bulk and strength to muscles. It is therapeutic because it adds water back to muscle cells. If you want to help maintain your muscles (you lose about 1 percent of body mass yearly after the age of 45), creatine supplementation can help.

If you're interested in trying creatine for yourself, it is widely available in powder or pill form at many health food or drug stores. Or, you can try my personal formulation, Ultimate Bionic Plus, and see for yourself how the right combination of muscle-supporting nutrition can keep you strong, toned and athletic. Not only does Ultimate Bionic Plus have the recommended daily dose of 2,000 mg of creatine, but it also contains six more muscle-supporting ingredients, all in a delicious drink mix. Read more about it on page 311 (See your Wellness Directory on page 410 for ordering information).

#2: Safeguard your prostate health, naturally

The history of using plant extracts to promote prostate health dates back to descriptions written on an Egyptian papyrus 15 centuries before Christ. The American Indians have been using saw palmetto (*Serenoa repens*) to support urinary tract health for centuries. And in Europe, it has been held in high regard for years.

Several studies about saw palmetto have been published in the last few years, and more research is cropping up all the time. All of them tout the prostate health boosting benefits of the free fatty acids in saw palmetto.

Research has shown that saw palmetto promotes prostate health by supporting healthy testosterone levels.

A 1996 study published in the medical journal *Prostate* found that saw palmetto promotes a strong and healthy urine flow.

In a trial reported in an issue of *Current Therapeutic Research*, 505 patients were given an oral preparation of saw palmetto, taking 160 mg twice daily.

Using no less than five means of comparison (the International Prostate Symptom Score, a quality-of-life score, urinary flow rates, residual urinary volume, and patient prostate size), the researchers showed that saw palmetto produced significant improvement after only 45 days of treatment.

After 90 days, 88 percent of the patients considered the therapy successful. Side effects were reported in only 5 percent of the patients in the three-month study.

No one knows exactly how saw palmetto works, but it definitely works—naturally promoting prostate health, with little or no serious side effects or adverse reactions!

Saw palmetto is just the beginning:

Saw palmetto isn't the only natural, plant-based solution that has been shown to be effective in protecting prostate health. Other extracts are commonly taken from the pygeum Africanum (African plum) and radix Urtica (stinging nettle) plants. The positive effects of these extracts are attributed to their phytosterols, steroid-like properties with a mild hormonal effect. Of the phytosterols, one of my favorites is sitosterol.

In a double-blind, placebo-controlled study published in the British medical journal *The Lancet*, patients treated with beta-sitosterol showed it promoted strong urinary flow and emptying of the bladder.

Even that old standby ginseng gets into the prostate act. It's an adaptogen (capable of many different functions). It adapts to the situation as needed. You're probably already familiar with the energizing and immune-boosting properties of ginseng. Well, ginseng has also demonstrated an ability to support your prostate!

Various vitamins and minerals may also contribute to overall prostate health. Vitamins C and E offer good antioxidant protection, and an amino acid "cocktail," made up of glycine, glutamine, and alanine can help support prostate health.

To read more about beta-sitosterol, see my report on page 133.

#3: Last, but certainly not least, let's talk about sex, my friend

We both know there's nothing quite like the feeling of showing your wife you've still got the goods. Yet so many men are having just "OK" sex... or no sex at all. That is NO way to live. But let me make one thing perfectly clear: it's NOT your fault.

All men should be doing something to promote healthy levels of PDE5 since PDE5 is the substance in your body responsible for shutting "things" down when you're finished with them.

But there are herbs that help promote healthy levels of PDE5 in your system—icariin and Cnidium monnieri. Both have been used around the world to help support full, strong erections. These gifts from nature give you the extra advantage you need to:

- **Support** rock solid erections

- **Satisfy your lover** with wild lovemaking she's been waiting for

- **Get the extra support you need** to have the time of your life in bed

Sound too easy? It almost IS too easy—but I'm certain you'll be blown away by your own bedroom performance (and so will SHE). And if you want a seriously intense extra boost, pop an extra dose an hour before getting randy.

If you're looking to get your hands on these two sexual helpers, look no further than your local drug store. But if you want to get two in one for a price that won't bust your wallet, try my **Ultra Turbo HG**.

Ultra Turbo HG works great when used with other natural performance products too—especially L-Arginine. That's because L-Arginine helps blood get to your member... and **Ultra Turbo HG** helps promote healthy levels of PDE5. (Ordering information can be found in the Wellness Directory on page 410.)

A thousand years of good, hard erections

For almost a thousand years, men in China, and India have used an herbal remedy derived from the puncture vine to help produce sustained erections. This incredible herb is **Tribulus terrestris Linn**.

Physicians in ancient India were the first to

recognize the plant's aphrodisiac properties and recommended its use in rejuvenating formulations. Researchers have even shown these properties.

T. terrestris Linn has been traditionally used to help support libido, and erections. T. terrestris Linn is rich in biologically significant components, saponins, flavonoids, alkaloids, oils, calcium, phosphorus, iron, and potassium.

T. terrestris Linn is available in some health-food stores.

A few words of caution

Exercise caution when deciding to supplement your hormone levels. Before you begin hormone supplementation, be sure to have your hormone levels tested by your physician. The effects of the long-term use of hormone supplements like ASD have not been thoroughly studied. I don't recommend using this powerful hormone in large doses. Small doses taken throughout the day can help bring your testosterone level up significantly, so large doses are unnecessary.

Get erect with these amino acids

If you're unable to get hard and stay that way, a deficiency of NO may be the cause. Nitric oxide (NO), which is not the same as nitrous oxide (or laughing gas), is a naturally occurring chemical resulting from the synthesis of the amino acid arginine. NO relaxes the smooth muscles of the penis and allows blood to more readily flood the tissues. Furthermore, recent research has shown that NO helps smooth-muscle tissues remain or become flexible, and it relaxes blood vessels, making it instrumental in fighting cardiovascular disease.

Meat, poultry, and eggs are prime sources of arginine—one more reason men shouldn't skimp on protein sources. Your body can make some arginine, but taking supplemental L-arginine can more quickly replenish your supply and provide more "food" to create greater quantities of nitric oxide. A study conducted at Harbor-UCLA Medical Center showed that L-arginine-laced water fed to rats for eight weeks increased NO levels (*Journal of Urology* 1997;158:942-7).

L-aspartic acid can help increase stamina and resist fatigue. In addition, it helps convert amino acids into usable compounds. By assisting with the conversion, it may more quickly convert arginine to nitric oxide, which means you could help increase your hardness, have more erections, or stay harder longer. Alfalfa sprouts are among the richest food sources of aspartic acid. Adding a handful of them to your next salad or sandwich might help bolster your system. If you'd rather take a supplement,

L-aspartic acid is available in capsule or powder form at most health-food stores.

Feeding your sex drive

Aphrodisiacs are usually thought of as herbal concoctions that supplement your diet to enhance libido and endurance. But you might be surprised to learn that some foods that you eat every day can also help you finish whatever you start.

Chocolate. Cocoa beans have long been revered as a way to create sexual desire and instill virility and endurance.

Despite its rich history, chocolate's effect on sensuality has been treated as nothing more than unsubstantiated hype. Whether or not mainstream medicine wants to acknowledge it, cocoa contains numerous components that produce positive moods and relieve negative feelings, including phenylalanine, an amino acid that replaces dopamine, which is a neurotransmitter associated with sexual pleasure and euphoria. Cocoa also causes your body to release beta phenylethylamine, a sexual stimulant and a mood enhancer.

Oysters. I told you earlier just how important zinc is for boosting your testosterone levels. Oysters are loaded with zinc and are a tasty way of keeping you fit and ready to perform!

Zinc is also essential for vaginal lubrication. As women age, natural lubrication diminishes. Eating oysters is an easy way to increase that natural moisture.

Caffeine. While everyone has told you to lay off the coffee because it'll stimulate you too much, maybe that's exactly what you need. Being stimulated is what sex is all about! Although you might have to take it in moderation, one cup of coffee could be just what you need to get your blood vessels dilated and blood rushing.

Celery. Who would have thought that celery would be a sex food? As it turns out, this unassuming vegetable contains androsterone, an important hormone that helps reinforce libido.

Strawberries. Strawberries contain a significant number of vitamins and minerals and 18 amino acids, including tryptophan and phenylalanine (mood enhancers), arginine (a precursor to the production of nitricoxide), and aspartic acid (an amino acid that helps your body use arginine in the production of nitric oxide). Besides the physical effect on your body, strawberries have another important element—color. Red is considered by most men and women to be symbolic of sex. The very image of popping a plump red berry in your mouth—or your partner's—has immense sensual appeal.

You need more sex!

Now that you've increased your testosterone levels to a decent level, and you've gotten your libido raging, here's a good way to put it to good use: more sex!

Researchers studied 918 men ages 45 to 59 for 10 years and found that men who had the most orgasms (averaging 100 per year, or about two per week) had a death rate 64 percent lower than that of men who had the fewest orgasms (less than one a month).

The basic premise here is that you've got to have sex. The old saying is true—if you don't use it, you'll lose it. To decrease your odds of contracting age-related illnesses, you should have an average of at least two orgasms a week. A Southern Illinois School of Medicine study showed that for migraines, an orgasm can be more effective than aspirin.

There are plenty of other studies that show sex is a life-lengthening endeavor. If you've been missing out on your regular dose of "vitamin S," here's some good ammo to help you get back in the saddle again.

A study out of Scotland reveals that people who have sex at least three times a week look 12 years younger than their out-of-action counterparts. During sex, the body's production of hormones is enhancing the body and mind, and increasing endorphins, thus acting as a veritable fountain of youth.

Chapter 15:

The Sexual Pitfall That Can Snare Any Man Over 50!

If your interest is waning, your confidence is fading and your sex life is on life support you must know—**there could be a specific villain at work**—and help is on the way.

In fact, there's a *little-known*, incredibly easy secret that helps you to ensure infinite sex and maintain masculine muscle mass—*no matter what your age*. And it all comes down to avoiding the gaping pitfall we can easily fall victim to. I call it the *"T-minus Condition."*

It's silent. It's sinister. And it can bury your sex drive six feet under. Even worse...

> **"By middle age and older, virtually all men experience it."**
>
> —Dr. Matthew Hoffman, contributing author for WebMD

You know it's bad when even the mainstream takes notice.

But this time, even they couldn't ignore it! The *T-minus Condition* is stripping men of their confidence, their strength, and all that it means to be a man.

I'm not here to remind you of long-gone machismo and swagger—but to show you the MANHOOD MIRACLE that helps boost the very essence of what makes you a man in the first place.

I've been tracking the *T-minus Condition*, along with its many age-related pitfalls, for decades. That means I'm constantly in search of the "manhood miracle" that can knock this condition down for the count and keep your masculinity at its peak.

Because with a secret like that in your hands you could *easily* be...

- Chasing your wife up the stairs because much to her disbelief—you're ready to go again!

- Giving her something to smile about with the performance of a lifetime.

- Looking like your youthful self with a firm body, a flashing smile and the sturdy swagger that'll catch more than your wife's attention.

Like I said, I call it the *T-minus Condition* and unfortunately—most men over 50 will experience it. It's when the MAN POWER substance in your body—testosterone—starts to tailspin down, down, down.

That can lead to... a lack of GUSTO, shrinking muscles, hair loss, a new "spare tire" on

Yawning may mean you're ready for sex!

Here's the latest theory on yawning—you're ready for sex. It seems that yawning and stretching in all males (animals and men) may be closely related to sexual arousal (*European Journal of Pharmacology*, 1998;343(1):1-16). Nitric oxide and the excitatory amino acids (e.g., aspartic acid) are at higher levels when you yawn and stretch.

The next time you yawn and stretch, don't go to sleep when you hit the sack. You'll want to take advantage of that excess nitric oxide. Excess amounts should be dispersed from your body, and sex is as good a way as any to channel it out.

your waist and apathy towards your favorite activity—all night sex.

When you need to stem the tides of the *T-minus Condition* (as most of us men over 50 do), you need a weapon that's... effective, powerfully potent, and natural.

In my search, anything with less than all three is tossed into the scrap pile—which is why until recently, I had come up plumb empty.

But a breakthrough discovery has been brought to my attention and I want to pass on the life-changing news to you first...

- It boasts libido and performance results that will have you racing to the bedroom to give it a whirl

- It increases natural free testosterone— the very substance that makes you a man, when combined with exercise

- It gives you the ability to support firm muscles and get BIGGER (*all* over) for the kind of manly confidence you'll feel in public and *certainly* in private

- And most importantly—this secret is as natural as the air you breathe

Are you intrigued? You should be...this could be all you need to hold on to every ounce of your masculinity—and make it grow and grow with each passing year.

Let me show you how this secret and the *T-minus Condition* work... with one simple question...

As you age through your 60's, 70's and beyond—do you want to be a Clint Eastwood... or a Woody Allen?

That should be an easy question. Many men (thanks to the T-minus Condition) get smaller, balder, weaker and just plain softer as the odometer ticks away.

But then you have men like Clint Eastwood. It's hard to believe he's 82-years-old. He still struts the red carpet with the same confidence and machismo that he had in his Dirty Harry days and heck——he has nearly the same physique.

The pitfall that kills your sex drive is declining levels of the substance that makes you a man. Mighty muscles, a surging manhood, and the *desire* (*and ability*) to please your wife over and over all start with the ultimate sex substance, **testosterone.**

A few lucky men have avoided the sex-draining pitfall without any help. For the rest of us, this secret has arrived that could give you...

The yowsa! sex you deserve!

In some regions of the world they call it *bockshorn*, literally meaning the "ram's horn."

It sounds like something you'd hear a Viking scream as he runs into battle... which is fitting because it is the most MANLY SECRET nature has to offer. It could catapult your libido to new heights.

It could have your wife demanding an encore... and shocked when you quickly deliver a repeat performance. It could keep you out of the sexual pitfall and increase levels of the very substance that made you the man you are today.

With this secret on your side imagine being stacked with...

BIG results, BIG MACHISMO, BIG everything you want!

It's always been the #1 complaint I hear from

men. So, for years, I've been searching for a way to combat the *T-minus Condition*. I've read a library's worth on diets, aphrodisiacs, exercise routines, and experimental "mojoboosters" that are just coming into the limelight.

And you know what I've found? *They are all bogus*.

They're either weaker than Don Knotts at an arm-wrestling contest or...

They're *unnaturally* strong—doing irreversible damage to the very parts of your body you're trying to help.

It's literally a game of testosterone tug-of-war. And for a while, it seemed like there wasn't any help on the horizon for the millions of men who need it.

Then something special happened...

I began to hear of a special clover found in remote portions of India that seemed to have an interesting relationship with testosterone. It was *the secret of the ram's horn*.

I know, I know—a *special clover*? You've heard that before—and so have I, over and over again...

But once I poured myself into the research, it wasn't the actual clover I was interested in—**it was the seeds that it produces.**

These puppies are loaded with one of the few substances I've ever found that along with exercise boost the essence of what makes you a man—safely and naturally.

They're called *saponin glycosides* and if you could bottle a pure extract of this stuff, **boy oh boy**—you could feel like a sexual superman... who could keep Lois Lane up all night long.

Finally, progress! But there was just one problem...

Sure, the ram's horn secret struck the perfect balance of sex-surging support, but to get the real kick-in-the-pants you want, you'd need to eat your weight in seeds.

So you might feel aroused, randy and capable... but probably too stuffed to do anything about it.

I thought it was *"back to the drawing board"*... but luckily for you, me, and every man over 50, a solution was already in the works...

With the writing on the wall, a group of scientists set out to harness the manpower found in the ram's horn secret. By carefully studying, growing and isolating the *saponin glycosides* found in these tiny seeds they were able to produce maximum results (and just wait until you see the results I'm talking about).

This is a special advancement in sexual health and I'm not waiting a moment longer to put the secret of the Ram's Horn to work for you. So today, I want to introduce you to what I consider...

The breakthrough formula every man must have: Ultimate Vigor

What if you could be... *more of a man*—and show her the difference? **Imagine,** more vigor coursing through your body. More masculinity propelling you to perform like a center-ring stud. More of the very essence of what makes you a man! Get ready—because that is the kind of potential hidden inside this **high-octane secret.**

This concentrated, *ready-to-rock-your-world* form of the ram's horn secret is called, *Testofen®.* So what's so special about this ingredient in my manpower breakthrough?

It's standardized to contain 50 percent of the ram's horn power source I told you about, *saponin glycosides.*

That's an incredibly potent amount and as you're about to see—I've made it even bolder!

But as you can imagine, with that much manpower, scientists were itching to take this breakthrough for a test run in the lab. It did not disappoint.

The creators of Testofen set out to determine how this breakthrough man-booster would affect the level of testosterone in men. They put it to the toughest test on 55 men (ages 21-50), using a double-blind, randomized, placebo-controlled study. In the beginning, blood samples were taken to measure starting point testosterone levels.

The 55 men were separated into 2 groups and then for 8 weeks, one group took a placebo and the other group took 600 mg of this breakthrough. Over the course of the trial both groups engaged in resistance exercises.

At the end of 8 weeks, blood was drawn again... and the results were in.

Both groups performed the same exercise routine—yet the group taking Testofen experienced a much larger increase in free testosterone levels!

Results like this only come around once in a lifetime!

And by combining this breakthrough with another signature sex secret it can help you keep...

• Rock-hard erections...

• An incredible "reload and repeat" recovery turn around and...

• The desire to carry your wife up the stairs and prove you've still got the goods...

This is HUGE news for you!

Research shows this supercharged secret safely boosts healthy levels of free testosterone— the very substance that makes sex possible in the first place!

It's like giving John Wayne *even more* of his gritty machismo to work with... It's like infusing Steve McQueen with *even more* sex-seducing confidence... It's like taking the lever that controls your vim and vigor and *cranking it to new levels!*

And let me tell you—that's just the beginning...

When she enticingly asks, "What in the world has gotten into you?" You'll know—THAT'S YOUR ULTIMATE VIGOR AT WORK.

Are you worried that your interest in sex has sailed out to sea and isn't coming back?

Don't be.

That's the second secret behind the ram horn's power...Boost your testosterone and increase your desire for "rock around the clock" sex.

What if you could have a whole new *libido renaissance?*

Fifty-four men participated in a study sponsored by the makers of Testofen that tested its ability to increase libido. These were healthy men age 50 and under involved in stable relationships.

In this placebo-controlled study, half of the participants took a formula that included 300 mg of Testofen along with zinc, vitamin B6 and magnesium for six weeks.

During the course of the study, participants answered a specially-designed questionnaire that objectively asked about different aspects of sexual experiences, fantasies, arousal, and quality of orgasm. The higher the score—the higher the sexual satisfaction.

After just 3 weeks, the Testofen group saw an increase in every area...

Arousal, sexual experience and quality of orgasm—they all reported improvement in the treatment group!

Sturdy strength, a swinging swagger and the feeling that you're still man enough to keep up with any of the boys—can all start by looking in the mirror

When you like what you see—you'll be ready to head straight to the bedroom for a perfect-score performance.

And when you wrap your arms around your wife and elicit *"oooo's"* and *"ahhh's"* over your strength—you'll both be up the stairs faster than a prairie fire with a tailwind.

So how can you maintain your strength through the years and keep your bedroom confidence soaring? Ultimate Vigor has just the help for you...

It just makes plain sense.

You want to keep firm arms... bulging legs... and a back that's strong enough to carry your wife up the stairs and straight into the bedroom?

Then help your body out!

Testosterone is the "original" muscle pumper. It helped you bulk up in your adolescence and it can help you stay fit, firm and ready for fun to this day.

With the Ram's Horn Secret—you can boost this muscle machine safely and naturally.

And while I'm not the biggest believer in gym memberships, this is the ultimate way to get noticeable results with your workout routines. Heck, all the "working out" you'll be doing in the bedroom might even do the trick...

I know... you hear the word *testosterone* and immediately your mind might jump to fathead baseball players jabbing each other with syringes in the locker room. **This secret is very different**. Those are anabolic steroids and I would never put my name anywhere near them. That's synthetic garbage that mimics testosterone to fit into your hormone receptors.

But what I'm talking about is supporting your body's natural capabilities to produce testosterone all on its own. It's natural, and it's Nature's way of helping combat the T-minus Condition.

It's called *free testosterone*. It's the testosterone naturally found in your bloodstream. It's not synthetic and it's found in your body at every point in life. It just decreases as you age—and, as I've shown you, that's where the ram's horn secret steps in to rally the troops.

During their 8-week trial, the makers of Testofen monitored the vitals of every subject. Heart rate, respiratory rate, blood pressure, body temperature, blood biochemistry, even the complex workings of the immune system—they were all watched with "eagle-eye" attention for any adverse effects.

On all areas, the vitals remained normal between the group of men taking a placebo and the group of men taking Testofen.

I'm even using a special form of *panax ginseng*. What makes this form so special? This panax ginseng extract comes from plants that have been growing for *six years*. Only then are they harvested—and the potential is monumental...

- At 1,800 mg doses, it can cause significantly more rigidity during erections

- It has been shown to promote greater satisfaction during sex

- This "more, more MORE" breakthrough has been used for centuries in Asian cultures and has been analyzed in over 28 sexual function studies

But just like the ram's horn secret, I demanded only the most potent form. So the 350 mg of panax ginseng in Ultimate Vigor is standardized to 8 percent ginsenosides—the secret substance that gives panax ginseng its BOOM.

But it's not done yet...

What do you need to put your sex life over the top? Surging energy, strong erections, *"ready when you are"* confidence?

Ultimate Vigor rockets them all between your sheets! Because I've also added Vitamin B1, B2, B3 and B5. Since each once is essential in the energy process for your cells, they may help you REV YOUR ENGINE, so you can burst out of the gates with power!

Everything about the sex sensation, **Ultimate Vigor** has been carefully thought out to bring you **stronger, longer sex.**

Your manhood can be surging with the latest breakthrough in boosting your testosterone!

Your swagger could be swinging when she's purring like a kitten after another all-night session.

Your body could stay strong and fit because it's charged with the *essence of what makes you a man!*

You're getting the highest quality at the perfect amounts, which will all result in a "big bedroom bang." (Ordering information can be found on page 410.)

Chapter 16:

Health Miracles for Women: How to Banish Breast Cancer, Osteoporosis, Menopausal Miseries, and More

For many years, I have been saying that people are misled by the false paradigm of "early detection of cancer leads to a cure." This mantra has been especially touted for breast cancer, with women being urged to get mammograms early and often and to examine their own breasts every month. The unfortunate fact, however, is that these methods of detection have not reduced the number of breast cancer deaths.

Silencing the self-exam shakedown

In 1997, the *Journal of the American Cancer Institute* published a study stating that even a vigorous program of instruction in breast self-examination is not successful in early detection of breast cancer or in reducing deaths.

People have no idea what they are feeling when they do a self-examination. It takes years of practice. Many doctors never master the technique. Besides, even if patients could be magically transformed into examining clinicians, by the time a tumor is large enough to be detected by self-examination, the cancer is very advanced.

The mammogram myth

Mammograms, like self-exams, can only detect tumors when they have reached a certain size—a size large enough to equal an advanced state of cancer. In addition, the very act of performing a mammogram may activate an otherwise quiescent and benign condition. I call it the "compression syndrome." To get good pictures, the radiologist must compress the breast, and the more he squeezes, the better the pictures. If he misses a tumor, he is subject to litigation, or at least embarrassment, so he squeezes away.

At the International Breast Cancer Screening Conference in Brussels, held in September 2000, Professor Michael Baum of University College Hospital in London confirmed what I have been saying all along:

"Thousands of women are being deceived by the national breast cancer program, because they are led to believe that early detection of cancer will save their breasts... This is not true." Up to half of all women with "early" breast cancer are having mastectomies that might later prove to be unnecessary, he said.

The problem comes with so-called ductal carcinomas—small, localized, very confined lesions that usually require no therapy. They can be closely monitored with no risk to the patient and may never have to be treated. Yet, women are misled and panicked into an unnecessary mastectomy.

An effective early detection alternative

Our bodies contain certain levels of a substance called anti-malignan antibody, or AMA. When cancer is present in the body, levels of AMA are elevated in nearly 100 percent of cases. When performed correctly, the AMAS test has false-positive and false-negative rates of less than one percent!

Results of the AMAS test alone cannot be used to diagnose the presence of disease, but it can be a significant tool to help doctors correctly detect cases of cancer where other procedures have fallen short.

To learn more about the AMAS test, contact Oncolab, Inc.: (800)9CA-TEST; www.oncolabinc.com.

Protect yourself from breast cancer with one powerful nutrient

One of the major keys to preventing breast cancer may be as simple as the soil your food grows in. Studies have shown that the selenium concentration in an area's soil has a strong correlation with the rates of cancer in that area. The more selenium, the less cancer is found.

For example, the Netherlands, Canada, Den-

mark, and Switzerland have the highest inci-
dences of breast cancer in the world. These
same countries also have very low selenium intakes. On the other side of the coin, Bulgaria
and Japan have the lowest breast cancer rates—
and the diets of the women living there are high
in selenium.

Since it is rather difficult to know whether
or not the soil where you live is selenium-rich,
and since the foods you buy in the supermarket
are grown all over the country, it's best to
take supplemental selenium. 200 mcg a day is a
safe amount. Selenium supplements are available
in most health-food and drug stores.

A high-quality multi-vitamin will also likely have all the selenium you need. If you pre-
fer a food source of selenium, try eating Brazil nuts. They're the richest natural source of
this vital nutrient.

Heart disease—a bigger threat than breast cancer

Breast cancer is cited as women's primary
health concern: One in nine women will be diagnosed with it in their lifetime. But there is an
even bigger threat to women's health—one that
is often overlooked, misdiagnosed, or thought
of as a primarily male problem. Myocardial in-
farctions—heart attacks—kill one of every two
women. That's more than all cancers combined!
Until recently, many doctors and patients have
been unaware of the prevalence of heart attacks
in women over 50.

When this information hit the news, the "experts" began treating heart disease with hormone replacement therapy (HRT). What they didn't realize is that standard HRT doesn't prevent heart attacks... it can actually double your risk! Standard HRT for women is based entirely on the use of synthetic estrogen and progesterone. These man-made hormones are not the same as the ones that occur naturally in women's bodies. And in addition to increasing the risk of heart attack, there is also strong evidence that they increase the risk of breast cancer.

While all of the synthetic estrogen HRT experimentation was going on—with dismal results—researchers virtually ignored another hormone essential to good health in both women and men—testosterone.

Testosterone: It's not just for men anymore

Ample research now indicates that testosterone is perhaps the most overlooked hormone. While women need a smaller proportion of testosterone than men, it is just as important to female health as it is to male. Testosterone improves blood flow to the heart in both sexes, reducing the risk of heart attack. And testosterone's benefits don't stop there.

Testosterone has anticoagulant properties, which means it helps protect against stroke. It also helps to regulate blood sugar, making it a potential treatment for diabetes. In addition, testosterone has been used effectively in treating osteoporosis and signs of aging.

And, as if all of this weren't enough, testosterone has also shown remarkable results in treating the most dreaded of female health concerns: breast cancer. In a study performed at the Baton Rouge Menopause Clinic, researchers treated 4,000 patients with a combination of estrogen and testosterone. Only one patient in every 1,000 was diagnosed with cancer by the end of the study: That's less than half the national average!

Testosterone won't keep you living forever, and it isn't a cure-all, but it may drastically improve the quality of your health. Having your levels tested is the first step. To find a doctor skilled in the use of natural hormones who can help you with testing and any necessary therapy, contact the American College for Advancement in Medicine at (800)532-3688, www.acam.org.

One important note: Make sure your doctor does not use methyl-testosterone—it has been shown to be harmful to the liver.

Managing menopause

Thanks once again to a barrage of media hype, menopause has become a dreaded time in most women's lives. The myths surrounding menopause are more dangerous than the experience itself: Women are conditioned to expect—and fear—a whole host of problems from weight gain to mood swings to depression to vaginal dryness. Most

of these symptoms have no connection—physi-
ologically—to menopause but are just normal,
natural changes to the aging female body.

Menopause does, however, have one symptom all
its own: Hot flashes. Hot flashes are related to
decreased estrogen, which is the primary complaint with menopause. They're uncomfortable,
yes, but bear in mind that hot flashes are not
dangerous, and using hormone replacement therapy to calm them is hardly worth the potential
negative side effects when there are a number
of other steps to take first.

The key to coping with hot flashes is not to
let them frighten you. Anxiety can actually
trigger an attack, so reducing stress can reduce the number of hot flashes you experience.

Next, reduce your alcohol intake. Alcohol
can trigger hot flashes in many women, so pay attention to your own reaction. If you have a hot
flash after you've had a drink, it's a good in-
dication that you may be sensitive to alcohol.

Several nutrients can help alleviate the discomfort of hot flashes. Bioflavonoids and vitamin
C have been used for over 30 years to reduce the
severity of hot flashes.

Chapter 17:

Health Miracles for Men: Real Prostate Solutions— Keeping Your Prostate Healthy for the Long Haul

When you talk about prostate trouble, you've put your finger on the classic definition of an "old man's disease." Chances are your grandfather suffered from prostate trouble, your father suffered from it, and even good old Uncle Ted suffered from it.

But you don't have to.

Believe it or not, all it takes is a few minutes a day to spare yourself the risk of doctor-caused impotence and incontinence and decades of inconvenience and embarrassment.

A swollen prostate: The biggest little problem plaguing most men

The prostate gland is a problem waiting to happen... right where you least want one. This little troublemaker is a one-inch, walnut-shaped gland that produces the liquid portion of semen. It occupies a very sensitive loca-

tion, surrounding the urethra just at the base
of the bladder. As such, it's a bull in a china
shop. Anything can go wrong.

One of the most common prostate problems is
swelling of the prostate gland. The prostate
simply grows larger over time. No problem—
until it's shoved against surrounding tissue.
Then it stops expanding outward and starts to
grow inward, clamping down on the urethra.

That's when the frustrating, often debilitating, and definitely humiliating symptoms begin: difficulty initiating a urine stream, a
weak, interrupted stream, embarrassing dribble,
and getting up several times during the night
to urinate. In severe cases, you may not be able
to urinate at all!

These symptoms—and their attendant fears of
incontinence and impotence—send thousands of
men running to the doctor every year. Unfortunately, most men run in the wrong direction,
right smack into the old medical 1, 2, 3:

1. Most prostate problems get treated by
   urologists.

2. Urologists are surgeons.

3. Surgeons don't get paid for not
   performing surgery.

The older you get, the higher your chances
are of dealing with this problem—especially if
you choose to do nothing about it now. It's a
fact that half of all 60-year old men are deal-

ing with prostate concerns. By 85, the number is as much as 90 percent.

What causes the prostate to swell?

No one knows for sure. The prostate's function is not yet fully understood. The most widely accepted theory is that it's linked to the chemistry of testosterone. As desirable as this hormone is for males, it is sometimes metabolized into dihydrotestosterone (DHT), a problematic steroid now widely believed to be responsible for the development of an enlarged prostate gland.

According to this theory, the swelling is caused by an accumulation of DHT. This potent hormone, which is believed to have twice as much impact per molecule as ordinary testosterone, is thought to cause an overproduction of cells, hence the enlargement of the prostate.

The conversion of testosterone into DHT is controlled by 5-alpha reductase, an enzyme manufactured by your body—but the conversion rate increases over time. By supporting healthy levels of this enzyme, it may be possible to protect the health of your prostate.

Your (flower) garden-variety prostate support

You might also protect your prostate by taking a pollen extract called Cernitin. Marketed as Cernilton®, this proprietary flower-pollen extract has anti-inflammatory properties and helps reduce fluid retention.

In one study, 70 men took 378 mg of Cernitin, 286 mg of a phytosterol/saw palmetto and beta-sitosterol complex, and 100 IU of vitamin E for 90 days, while another group of 57 men took a placebo. After 12 weeks, the group taking Cernilton experienced a more restful night's sleep (Family Practice News 1999; 29(22):24).

You can buy Cernilton from Graminex in Saginaw, Michigan. Their product is called Prostanex. Call (877)472-6469 or visit Graminex on the Internet at www.graminex.com. A bottle of 90 tablets retails for $39, and the recommended dose is three tablets daily.

The big Z:
The last word in prostate care

Still more good news for keeping your prostate healthy comes straight off the periodic table of elements.

Testosterone is closely interrelated with the mineral zinc. This mineral could help promote healthy levels of testosterone. The prostate also just happens to be the organ where zinc is stored in great abundance!

Zinc plays an important role on the health of your prostate. Did you know your semen has 36 times more zinc than your blood? Supplements of zinc have been shown to be useful in supporting male fertility. Since healthy zinc levels can promote healthy levels of testosterone, it is possible that zinc can support your sex drive. Low levels of zinc can also lead to a loss of appetite.

Sex is good for you—have more of it!

Sex has a number of benefits aside from the obvious. It has been shown to increase circulation to all parts of the body, lower cholesterol levels, reduce stress, relieve pain, boost immune function, improve cognitive function, promote bone growth, and improve the quality of sleep.

Frequent sex actually tones and protects your plumbing, and research has even shown that sexually active men have fewer prostate problems and gain added protection from testicular and prostate cancer.

It is essential to supplement your diet with zinc. The usual recommended dosage for adults is 30 mg daily. Doses of up to 50 mg a day are considered safe, but doses higher than 50 mg are not recommended and could have an adverse effect on health. Doses of 150 mg or greater can cause diarrhea. Zinc is also found in food sources such as whole grains, most seafood, sunflower seeds, soybeans, and onions.

Pumpkin seeds are a balanced source of zinc and magnesium, another mineral shown to have positive benefits on the prostate. Pumpkin seeds also provide essential fatty acids (EFAs). EFAs are closely associated with the health of the prostate gland, particularly since EFAs are the nutritional precursors to prostaglandins, which, in turn, inhibit testosterone from binding to the prostate.

And finally, lycopene is a fat-soluble carotenoid with antioxidant properties that support prostate health.

There have been a number of studies on lycopene, including one at Harvard that followed 47,000 participants, all pointing toward lycopene's prostate health-boosting properties.

Traditional cancer solutions— modern day bloodletting?

Someday, people will look back at today's conventional cancer treatments and consider them as crude and barbaric as we view the medieval practice of bloodletting today.

Chemotherapy is perhaps the most common mainstream cancer solution. Although it can be helpful in cases of testicular cancer and lymphocytic leukemia, chemotherapy is basically fraudulent and illogical. How in the world can oncologists think they are treating rationally when their so-called therapy is destroying the immune system?

Sure, the tumor may shrink—its immunity is being attacked as well as yours. So it becomes a race as to which will kill the patient first: the cancer or the treatment? The chemicals, although they kill the rapidly dividing cancer cells the fastest, also kill healthy cells in the body. And the cure rate is dismal at best.

The McGill Cancer Center in Canada, one of the largest and most prestigious cancer treatment centers in the world, did a study of oncologists to determine how they would respond to a diagnosis of cancer. On the confidential questionnaire, 58 out of 64 doctors said that all chemotherapy programs were unacceptable to them and their family members. The overriding reasons for this decision were that the chemotherapy drugs are ineffective and that they have an unacceptable degree of toxicity. These are the same doctors who will tell you that their chemotherapy treatments will shrink your tumor and prolong your life!

Surgical removal of the cancerous tumor offers yet another dangerous option for cancer patients. When the malignant tumor is removed, normal, healthy tissue is often removed as well—and the process weakens the immune system and other systems in the body that are essential for resisting disease. For men, surgery is often used in the case of prostate cancer to remove testicles. Even if the cancer may be stopped, impotence is often the result.

Don't allow mainstream medicine to brainwash you into thinking that their way is the only way.

CLA curbs the spread of cancer

Animal research has shown that conjugated linoleic acid (CLA) stops the spread of human prostate cancer cells. After rats were injected with cancer cells, they were divided into groups fed CLA, linoleic acid (LA), and a diet with no additives. After eight weeks, the mice eating CLA-spiked feed had a significantly reduced number of tumors. The CLA-fed mice also experienced a unique phenomenon—tumor growth progressed as expected for five to six weeks and then started to die, leaving nothing but a scar as a reminder of the former tumor's presence.

The purpose of the study was to determine if CLA could stop the prostate cancer cells from spreading to the lungs. Eighty percent of the control group and 100 percent of the LA group showed lung-cancer metastasis.

Only 10 percent of those in the CLA group had started growing tumors in their lungs by the

The seedy side of life

A study showed that men ages 53 to 74 with low-grade prostate cancer reduced the proliferation of their cancerous cells by consuming 30 grams of flaxseed over a period of 21 to 43 days (Family Practice News 1999; 29(22):24).

If you do any woodwork or furniture refinishing, you already know about flaxseed as an ingredient in linseed oil. If you've been making your own linseed oil to preserve a nice finish on wood, divert some of the flaxseed to your plate. Flaxseed is available at health-food stores and most major grocery stores.

end of the study (Anticancer Research 1998;18 (3A):1429-34).

CLA may also help reduce body fat. In lab experiments, CLA-fed rats showed reduced quantities of fatty deposits on their livers after being fed a CLA-enriched diet for two weeks. Urine tests indicated that the rats were passing ketones, which is indicative of weight loss by burning fat (Lipids 1999;34(9): 997-1000).

The participants in the above studies were fed a one percent solution of CLA. This equates to approximately three 1,000 mg doses per day for the average person. If you're a big man, or if you are extremely active physically and eat much more than the average person, you might want to increase that dosage. CLA should be available at your local health-food store.

Enhance your sexual performance while fighting cancer

Scientists are finding that DHEA not only boosts sexual performance, but could play an important role in fortifying your immune system for a longer, more energetic life by counteracting the stress hormone cortisol.

Most spectacularly, researchers at the University of Mississippi Medical Center demonstrated that doses of DHEA regulated growth of prostate tumors in mice, while at the same time boosting their sex drives!

DHEA formulations are available in most health-food stores. However, since DHEA is a hormone, you should work closely with a doctor if you decide to pursue this therapy. For a referral to a physician in your area skilled in alternative medicine, please contact the American College for Advancement in Medicine at (800)532-3688 or www.acam.org.

Chapter 18:

One Pill in the Palm of Your Hand—And Your Prostate Protection is Set!

I'm going to let you in on a secret—but I have to warn you—if you're currently gulping down handfuls of pills and paying through the nose to support your prostate health, maybe take a seat first.

You see, there is a way you can help:

1. Keep a POWER STREAM flowing...

2. Drain your bladder dry with ease...

3. And sleep more soundly—so you can be raring to go come sunrise...

All for <u>HALF the price and in JUST ONE TINY PILL</u>!

Think I'm yanking your chain? Then you just haven't been introduced to...The One Pill Powerhouse! This is the secret "scheming vitamin hucksters" are scrambling to keep from you! And it's not hard to see why...

Heck, the star nutrient's amazing power has been published in *The Lancet*...

It's been shown to support strong urinary flow by over 372 percent when compared to a placebo. And that prominent study revealed it could promote complete bladder emptying by over 200 percent when compared to a placebo!

Now I might sound like a broken record here, but it can do all this for half the price of saw palmetto.

Frankly, I just want to shake the greed out of these "fat cat" formulators telling you that you need up to 6 pills a day for prostate protection. They darn well know you have a better option!

My breakthrough could cut your nightly trips with just one pill...for less than a dollar a day.

Imagine, you spring out of bed, refreshed, ready to take on your day—because you didn't get up once the night before...or the night before that...

You march out in the kitchen and instead of lining up 6 horse pills along the counter and mentally prepping yourself for a torturous routine. You pour one, easy-to-swallow pill into the palm of your hand—and you get all of the protection that I've mentioned above—for half the price of most other formulas you'll find.

That is the power of my prostate formula,

Ultimate PRO Support—it has everything you need...and nothing you don't.

But how is it possible? How can I give you premium prostate support without sending the price through the roof? The secret lies with the hero behind many of today's most effective solutions...

Here's the REAL superstar that gives those expensive prostate herbs their power

The magic bullet behind all 3 prostate herbs is a powerful plant compound called: Beta Sitosterol. It's actually a powerful kind of phytosterol—and is similar to cholesterol.

After reviewing three major studies on beta sitosterol, I was consistently amazed by its effectiveness: Not only can it help boost the power of your urinary flow; it can also dramatically lower the amount of urine left in your bladder.

That means you won't have to get up every 5 minutes during the night and run to the bathroom. Imagine that? Night after night of restful sleep!

Now, I know what you're thinking... If beta sitosterol is all you really need, then why bother with saw palmetto in the first place? Well, some manufacturers are making lots of money from prostate herbs.

Here's the problem: The price and availability

of true saw palmetto is always fluctuating. This leaves the door open to unscrupulous vendors.

Cheap saw palmetto supplements may be enticing, but as you are well aware, you get what you pay for. (That's why I insist on paying top dollar for the saw palmetto I do recommend. But the best saw palmetto means you'll pay a higher price for prostate support.) But...

You can save yourself a TON of money—and bypass the need for herbs altogether!

Think of it this way: For all these years, scientists have been scouring the earth, looking for herbs that contain and deliver beta sitosterol. So far, the most effective herbs are the popular "Big 3": pygeum, pumpkin seed and world-renowned saw palmetto.

But why should you pay big prices for exotic herbs in pricy prostate supplements when you can get the real deal for half the price?

Let's cut to the chase—You don't need expensive herbs to protect your prostate. And I don't care if those fly-by-night pill pushers come after me for telling you!

My prostate breakthrough Ultimate PRO Support, gives you EVERYTHING you need—and leaves OUT all the expensive extras.

Many studies have shown: beta sitosterol can help relieve the stress of your nagging prostate.

When doctors do research, they usually start with a meta-analysis. That means we do a study of all the studies—an overview of everything out there. Well, that's what I started.

I knew beta sitosterol was a more affordable option—without sacrificing effectiveness. But I wanted to get to the bottom of it...

And boy-oh-boy did I turn up some impressive evidence.

In 1995, a groundbreaking study was published in the British medical journal *Lancet*. They used something called the **International Prostate Symptom Score** to measure various facets of urinary flow, like the strength of urine flow and residual urine left in your bladder. (You know how scientists love to measure everything...)

Well, they studied 200 men. One hundred received beta sitosterol and 100 got a placebo (dummy pill).

After 6 months, the men who took beta sitosterol:

- Showed a dramatic improvement on their International Prostate Symptom Score—an amazing 50 percent improvement!

- Strengthened their urinary flow by 53 percent!

- Reduced the level of residual urine in their bladder by 54 percent!

- Maintained ALL the benefits of their treatment after an 18-month follow up!

I hear stories of men getting up 4... 5... 6 times a night—just to

stand over the toilet and wait...

Just take John K. from Richmond, Virginia. He wrote in to say: "I was going to the bathroom 2 or 3 times during the night and more often during the day."

Sound familiar?

Most men hope that prostate trouble will pass them by. But the numbers tell a different story. One out of two American men get hit by the time they're 50. And by the time you reach your 80s, your chances are at about 80 percent!

But there's no need to stay up at night worrying once your doctor has checked you out and told you that this is just a part of growing older...

The powerful, natural ingredients in Ultimate PRO Support can help relieve your anxiety—and helps keep you in control.

Ultimate PRO Support puts your mind at ease from worries like:

Standing over the toilet—with NOTHING happening...

Dribbling and dribbling, never able to fully empty your bladder...

A weak stream, with the never-ending starts and stops...

The urge to go more at night—getting out of bed 3, 4, 5 times or more...

Even if Ultimate PRO Support had just one
ingredient—the remarkable and affordable beta
sitosterol—it would still be your best bet for
long-term prostate health.

But I didn't stop there...

Super-charge YOUR manhood!

Ultimate PRO Support has 4 prostate and sexual health supporters for 4 TIMES the protection...

Your prostate is an important part of your
"male plumbing." It's where most of your semen
is made. And here's the real kicker: Without a
healthy prostate, you can't have a REAL ejaculation!

(The contractions of your prostate move semen through your urethra during ejaculation...
So maintaining a healthy prostate is essential
to a healthy sex life!)

Men from every state in the union write to
me asking me about the sexual side effects of
prostate trouble. That's why I packed Ultimate
PRO Support with potent doses of 4 essential
"man building" nutrients and minerals:

Zinc—70 percent of American men don't get
the recommended 11 mg of zinc per day. And that
can spell trouble. Your semen has 36 times more
zinc than your blood—and your prostate has the
highest concentration of zinc in your body.
(See the sexual connection?)

Zinc is a real "man's mineral." A healthy

level of zinc:

- Helps promote healthy levels of testosterone

- Could help in regulating how testosterone is secreted through your body.

Ultimate PRO Support delivers a full 25 mg of zinc in 3 easy-to-absorb forms. (Which is good news—many supplement forms of zinc cause queasiness and upset stomach. But with Ultimate PRO Support you NEVER have to worry.)

Vitamin E—You've probably heard a lot about the power of vitamin E. It's one of the most effective and versatile antioxidants on the planet. Together with beta sitosterol, vitamin E targets dangerous free radicals and provides your prostate with a shield of protection—sheltering it from the ravages of aging, oxidation and external threats.

Dozens of studies over the last two decades show the remarkable power of vitamin E and its ability to help promote a healthy prostate for a lifetime. It does this by supporting healthy prostate cell growth, helping to keep androgens (hormones) from negatively affecting your cells.

Vitamin E gives your manhood a boost too! Vitamin E promotes proper blood flow to the genitals, which is critical for supporting strong erections. Plus, vitamin E seems to have a protective effect on your body's formation of sex hormones, like testosterone.

Ultimate PRO Support gives you an ample supply of vitamin E (100 IU)—more than enough to give you double-barreled protection: For both your prostate AND your sex life!

Lycopene—If you've been watching the news lately, you may have seen the reports linking lycopene and prostate health. And they're all true! In fact, one study from Harvard University revealed that men who frequently ate foods high in lycopene lowered their risk of prostate health issues by up to 45 percent!

Lycopene is a carotenoid that gives tomatoes their red color. Its antioxidant power is double than most—and 100 times stronger than vitamin E! And its link to your prostate is undeniable.

Unless you really love tomatoes—like 5 or more large ones a day—I recommend you let Ultimate PRO Support supply you with the additional prostate protecting power lycopene can give you—Every day!

Selenium—Finally, I've included what I call every man's "must-have mineral." Its power to support your immune system is remarkable. And it's especially helpful for your prostate. As with lycopene, studies consistently show that men with higher levels of selenium have healthier prostates.

These days, getting selenium from your diet is harder and harder. That's why supplementing is so important. Minerals like selenium come from the soil. But strong fertilizers and commercial farming practices eliminate these minerals making it hard for you to get your daily supply.

Ultimate PRO Support gives you an extra shot of selenium, ensuring you're armed with one of the most powerful, prostate-friendly antioxidants ever discovered.

By now, I'm sure you can see how Ultimate PRO Support makes maximum prostate support a sure thing—at less than half the cost of other prostate formulas!

After all, why should the best prostate support cost more than your monthly telephone bill?! Ultimate PRO Support gives you maximum prostate protection AND supports a healthy sex life... ALL for less than a dollar a day!

Ultimate PRO Support ALREADY works for thousands of men, just like you—EVERY DAY! Now it's YOUR turn! (Go to page 410 for ordering information.)

Chapter 19:

Three Reasons You Don't Need "Regular" Prostate-Cancer Screening

---

I'm not usually a fan of *The New York Times*, but for once, they almost got a bit of health reporting right: An article published in *The Times* in May finally stated that the prostate specific antigen (PSA) test for prostate cancer doesn't work and sometimes is worse than nothing. Well, the article didn't exactly say it in those words, but it came close enough:

"A man's score on a routine blood test for prostate cancer fluctuates naturally over time, so doctors should repeat the test in four to six weeks before performing a biopsy, a new study has concluded." This is *The New York Times'* way of spinning the story—aided and abetted by the medical profession—so that people won't stop trusting the PSA altogether.

Here's the REAL scoop:

In a study of about 1,000 men, more than 20 percent were found to have elevated levels of prostate-specific antigen (PSA). But for half of those men, the level fell back to normal in subsequent tests.

The truth is the PSA test is so unreliable that it shouldn't be used at all. It leads to tens of thousands of unnecessary biopsies that are themselves inaccurate.

Biopsy needles can miss cancer tissue altogether, i.e., a "false negative." And if the initial results are negative, the doctor won't do a repeat biopsy—unless the PSA test is very high. But if a biopsy comes back positive, gets repeated, and the second result turns out to be negative, then where are you? Everybody is in confusionville, which is just short of disasterville.

So, the reasoning goes, "Let's take the prostate out—better safe than sorry." Well, you might be <u>very</u> sorry. You may become impotent, the surgery may spread the cancer, and you may have to wear Pampers for the rest of your miserable life. The operation is unnecessary in early cases of prostate cancer because most men outlive the cancer as they are very slow- growing <u>unless disturbed by a surgeon</u>. Autopsies have shown that a high percentage of elderly men die of other causes and never knew they had prostate cancer because they <u>stayed away from doctors</u>.

Actions to take:

(1) Don't submit to a needle biopsy. Remember, biopsies are one of the golden eggs of surgery—they're profitable, take little time to perform, and are relatively safe as far as <u>immediate</u> complications are concerned,

meaning a low liability risk for the surgeon. But experiments have demonstrated that after sticking a needle into cancer tissue, <u>cancer cells can be found in the bloodstream</u>. Where do the cancer cells "released" by biopsies go? It's not at all unlikely that they could manifest themselves in the bone and show up 10 years later as an incurable form of the disease.

(2) Don't waste your time with the PSA test either. It's been documented numerous times that early detection of prostate cancer via the PSA test doesn't translate into increased survival rates.

(3) If you're worried about cancer and feel like you've got to take some sort of test to evaluate your risk, instead of getting a PSA test, get a blood test called the AMAS—the Anti Malignin Antibody Screen. This test is the best by far as a screen for cancer anywhere in your body.

The test itself couldn't be easier. Your doctor simply takes a blood sample and sends it to a qualified lab where it is screened for Anti-Malignan Antibody (AMA), a naturally occurring antibody whose levels become elevated in the presence of cancer cells. These serum levels tend to rise early in the course of the disease, which means that you can detect the presence of cancer as much as several months—even a year—before other clinical tests find it.

The AMAS test can detect early cancer cells of all types (not just prostate cancer). It has an accuracy rate of greater than 95 percent. With a second test, the accuracy is greater than 99 percent. False positive (and false negative) rates are less than 1 percent.

Results of the AMAS test alone cannot be used to diagnose the disease. However, it is a remarkable breakthrough for the detection of cancerous cells, which, taken in conjunction with other factors, may help physicians arrive at a more concrete—and accurate—diagnosis. For more information on the AMAS test, contact Oncolab Inc. at (617)536-0095 or visit www.amascancertest.com.

(4) If the diagnosis is positive, don't let your physician rush you into surgery. Most cancers are slow-growing, and you need not panic into treatment. (The unfortunate fact is that if a tumor is fast-growing, mainstream therapies like chemotherapy and radiation will most likely be useless anyway.)

Chapter 20:

Reality Check:
The Extreme Dangers of Hormone Replacement Therapy

I know I've never had to go through menopause, but it doesn't take too much imagination to know that any potential relief from the symptoms of menopause can't possibly be worth the higher rates of ovarian cancer, higher rates of breast cancer, and higher rates of stroke that go along with hormone replacement therapy.

But hey, you can't have hot flashes when you're dead, right? And that's just how you could end up if you decide to take HRT.

In what could be the final nail in the coffin of HRT, the *Journal of the American Medical Association* published a report with the most damning evidence to date:

Women who take hormone replacement pills are <u>twice as likely</u> to die from breast cancer

This flies in the face of the former "prevailing thought"... the boneheaded notion that even though these pills could increase your risk of breast cancer, it was the type of cancer that would be "favorable and not much of a problem."

Really? People actually buy that line of B.S.?

They must. Because Big Pharma is still raking in billions with these cancer-causing concoctions.

But when Dr. Rowan Chlebowski of the Los Angeles Biomedical Research Institute analyzed data on more than 12,000 women from the Women's Health Initiative Study, he found that, compared to women who took placebo, twice as many women taking HRT died from breast cancer.

He also found that the women who developed breast cancer and who had taken HRT were 50 percent more likely to have their cancer spread to the lymph nodes than the women who took a placebo.

Given the latest information—plus the years of negative research that came before it—you'd think doctors would start looking for alternatives. Instead, they're only looking for excuses. Why else would they continue prescribing the stuff and think that simply lowering the dose is going to be any safer?

Has there been any research proving that fact? No!

But here's what research has proven...

- A study in the *Archives of Internal Medicine* found that women taking HRT are 21 percent more likely to develop kidney stones.

- A study in the *Lancet* found that HRT increased lung cancer deaths.

- And as you may recall, researchers had to pull the plug early on the Women's Health Initiative study because of the staggering increase in the risk of breast cancer, heart attack, and stroke.

I'm not opposed to hormone replacement therapy—you just need to make sure you're taking bioidentical hormones. Bioidentical hormones are made from natural substances within a woman's body—as opposed to Big Pharma's version, which comes from horse estrogens.

All of research shows that bioidentical hormones are safer and more effective than patentable molecules. They have fewer side effects. They can reduce the risk of heart disease, Alzheimer's disease, and breast cancer. They can improve memory, concentration, mood, and sleep patterns. The list goes on.

The evidence on the benefits of bioidentical hormones—and on the dangers of synthetic hormones—is hard to ignore, but the FDA is doing a darn good job doing just that.

They're so squarely in Big Pharma's camp that they're doing their best to help take out bioidentical hormones bit by bit. Case in point...

FDA takes aim at bioidentical hormone replacement therapy

Nurses in Oregon are currently fighting a bat-

tle to protect their right to prescribe the bioidentical estrogen hormone estriol... despite
the fact that mainstream's meds are killing
women at "twice the usual mortality rate,"—and
despite the fact that the FDA can't substanti-
ate a single adverse event for estriol.

Estriol's crime? It's not approved by the
FDA.

Hello! Of course it's not! It's a natural
substance found in women's bodies! Since when
did we need FDA approval for that? (Seems like
someone's getting too big for his britches!)
Besides, do you know how much money it costs to
get that "coveted" (and I use that term loose-
ly) stamp of approval? Upwards of $1 billion!
A non-patentable substance can't bring in that
kind of dough—and no company is going to spend
that kind of money on a substance they don't own
the rights to.

Regardless, Big Pharma must feel pretty
threatened by this little substance. Why else
would the company file a petition to have it
banned from the market? They shouldn't have had
a leg to stand on, but in the end, the only
thing that stopped the FDA from approving it
was the huge public outcry.

I know that the symptoms of menopause can be
unbearable. But the bottom line here is that
you don't have to put your life on the line to
find some relief. Contact a doctor who will work
with you to prescribe bioidentical hormones
that are right for you—at the right dose.

To find a doctor who will work with you to find a natural solution, contact the American College for the Advancement of Medicine at www.acamnet.org, or by calling (800) 532-3688.

Chapter 21:

7 "Forbidden" Foods You Should Eat Every Day

You've heard it said over and over again: "Meat and fat are bad! They'll clog your arteries and make you gain ungodly amounts of weight! If you value your life, you'll cut them from your diet!"

You'd think we were eating food laced with arsenic the way we've been told for the past 20 years to stay away from eggs, dairy products, and meat. And undoubtedly, after the millionth time or so, the message starts to sink in. The problem is, all this anti-meat, anti-fat propaganda is pure junk medicine.

Shed your spare tire in two weeks eating steak and eggs!

The truth is, you can eat all you want of the foods you love, lose weight, have more energy, and be healthier. So, go ahead, have a thick steak for dinner. And enjoy your bacon and three-egg omelet for breakfast!

Humans need the nourishment and satisfaction

of these high-protein, high-fat meals for good health. Forget what you've been told: Contrary to popular belief, fat does not make you fat! I've seen patients lose 50 pounds or more on a strict meat and fat diet. The real problems are the sugar and carbohydrates people eat along with the fat. For true good health, more energy, and real, permanent weight loss, you need to realign your eating machine, ditch carbohydrates like pasta salad and bran muffins, and knock sugar off its pedestal.

The no-good, low-fat diet

The USDA food pyramid nutrition recommendations are dead wrong. According to the food pyramid, carbohydrates should be consumed in greater quantity than any other nutrient while fat and protein should be consumed in smaller amounts. But there's proof that the pyramid needs to be reversed.

The popular trend of "carb loading"—stuffing yourself with bread, pasta, fruit, potatoes, etc.—is not the booster of health and athletic performance it has been made out to be. A study performed in South Africa showed that cyclists following a diet that included only 7 percent carbs could pedal twice as long as those on a 74 percent carb diet.

A Brazilian study found that increasing protein intake and decreasing carbohydrate intake increased energy and gave a definite nutritional and biochemical advantage to exercising rats. Rats receiving a high-protein diet had energy levels over three times as high as those of control groups and groups of rats placed on high-carb diets.

Why does eating more protein and fewer carbs actually help you?

By stripping carbohydrates from your diet, you will experience dramatic weight loss (even if other diets never worked for you), never be hungry, and improve your health... while continuing to eat and enjoy the foods you need to be healthy.

When you eat carbohydrates (breads, starches, and simple sugars), your body easily absorbs them and converts them into glucose in your blood—thus raising your blood-sugar levels. As a result, the hormone insulin is then produced to convert the glucose into fuel to run the body. However, when insulin appears on the scene to tell the body to burn glycogen, it also tells it to stop burning fat, and it stuffs the fat back into storage. And you know what it looks like there!

In addition, if you consume more carbs than you need for immediate energy, insulin converts the glucose into fat and puts this into storage as well. The glucose builds up day after day in your arteries (and in that spare tire) until your circulation is blocked, your tissues don't get nourished, and you end up with obesity, high blood pressure, cholesterol buildup, diabetes, heart disease, fatigue, impotence, or even cancer.

A diet based on meat and animal fats stabilizes blood sugar levels and turns your body from a sluggish carbohydrate burner into a fat-burning machine. It delivers the metabolic edge you need to protect yourself from the life-threatening conditions mentioned above. And it does so on the strength of protein!

Eat fat, get thin

As early as 1960, nutritionists noticed that the body uses stores of body fat—as opposed to carbohydrate fuel—for energy when carbohydrates are restricted. They were surprised by their patients' weight loss even in the presence of large amounts of dietary fat.

In a 1963 landmark weight-loss study, Dr. A. Keswick and G.L.S. Pawan, of London's Middlesex Hospital Medical School, found that mice on a high-protein (carb-restricted) diet used their own fat stores as fuel and lost weight, while mice on a high-carb diet used the carb's sugary fuel as energy and kept their fat (*Metabolism*, 1964).

Contemporary wisdom says that a diet rich in fats increases your risk of colorectal cancer, but Belgian researchers found that the risk of rectal cancer was doubled—not by fats—but by a high-carbohydrate diet.

They studied the eating habits, particularly fat intake, of over 3,500 subjects (*Nutrition and Cancer*, 1987). Even the control group had a higher incidence of cancer than the group on a high-fat diet!

A low-fat diet
can endanger your heart

A study reported in the *Journal of the American Medical Association* showed that aggressively restricting your fat intake may do more harm than good. The study looked at 444 men who had high levels of LDL ("bad" cholesterol). Many of the participants also had high levels of triglycerides, another indicator of bad heart health.

These men were separated into four groups, with the overall daily caloric intake from dietary fat being 30 percent, 26 percent, 22 percent, or 18 percent. Tests done one year later showed those on the least restrictive diet actually saw their LDL levels drop more than those on the other three regimens.

The more restrictive diets showed no additional benefit in other areas of health, such as weight, blood sugar, insulin, or blood-pressure levels. In fact, the two most restrictive diets ended up causing a decrease in HDL ("good" cholesterol) and an increase in triglyceride levels.

All that self-denial, and these poor guys were worse off than when they started.

Diabetic? Have a steak

I get a lot of flak for advocating red meat, but researchers at Purdue University and Penn State have found that fat in red meats and cheeses may prevent diabetes.

Their study found that conjugated linoleic acid (CLA), a polyunsaturated fatty acid found in meat, cheese, poultry, and eggs (all of the previously "exiled" foods), prevents the onset of diabetes in laboratory animals.

This suggests that CLA may help normalize or reduce blood-glucose levels and prevent diabetes. The researchers say that natural CLA appears to work as well as a new class of diabetes-fighting drugs, the thiazolidinediones (TZDs).

The research was conducted on a special breed of rat called the Zucker diabetic fatty rat, whose obesity and glucose intolerance mimics

Want to lose weight? Have another cup of real java

A recent study indicates that caffeine, when combined with carnitine and choline, decreases body fat and serum-leptin (blood fat) levels at a rate similar to mild exercise. While supplementing with this combination won't improve your cardiovascular fitness, it could give you that extra edge if you're trying to lose weight. If you need to reduce your triglyceride levels, then these three supplements will give you another advantage, as the study participants had significantly reduced triglyceride levels, whether they exercised or not (Journal of Nutrition 2000;130(2):152-7).

human adult-onset diabetes (also called type II, or noninsulin-dependent diabetes, the most common form of the disease). The rats were given doses of CLA for two weeks. At the end of the experiment, all of the control rats had developed diabetes and none of the rats on CLA had developed the disease.

Previous studies with CLA have shown that it can prevent the onset of certain cancers and reduce skin and stomach tumors in laboratory animals.

CLA is available as a dietary supplement in health food stores, but you should be advised that there is no toxicology data for it yet. A small percentage of thiazolidinedione patients have reported liver abnormalities, and human trials on CLA's effect on diabetes are set to begin soon.

Putting some specific foods under the nutrition microscope

Now that I've cleared up some of the misconceptions about the macronutrients—proteins, fats, and carbohydrates—I'd like to tell you the REAL truth about some specific foods you've been told were bad for you.

Coconut oil—a perfect food

Thirty years ago, the saturated fat vs. unsaturated fat debacle began—and coconut oil was cast out with the rest of the saturated fats as health-destroying scourges.

But the fact of the matter is that saturated fats, including coconut oil, are good for you. It's actually the unsaturated oils that do the most harm, causing cancer, heart disease, and obesity. Rather than contributing to excess weight, coconut oil has the unique ability to keep you lean.

Over 50 years ago, farmers began looking for a cheaper way to fatten their livestock. Coconut oil seemed an obvious choice, being much cheaper than grain, and since it was a type of fat, they figured that it made for fatter cows. Much to their surprise and dismay, the coconut-oil fed animals stayed lean, despite the fact that they consumed as much as, if not more than, grain-fed cows.

While skinny cows don't make for happy cattle farmers, thinner people make for a healthier population, and coconut oil can help achieve that. In addition to helping control weight, natural coconut oil acts as an antihistamine and also has anti-diabetic and anticancer properties.

And perhaps the best thing about coconut oil (as if all this weren't enough)? It has an amazing shelf life: It can be left at room temperature for over a year without becoming rancid!

Beer—toast to your health

The health benefits of beer are enormous. While it's composed mostly of water and alcohol, beer is often called "the complete food." It has a wide range of amino acids, proteins, polypeptides, and minerals, including potas-

Getting the most from the foods you eat

In the 1930s, Dr. Paul Kouchakoff, a researcher at the Institute of Clinical Chemistry, studied how cooked foods affect our bodies. Dr. Kouchakoff found that the higher the food's temperature, the greater the body's immune response. In other words, our bodies react to cooked foods the same way they react to foreign invaders:

They release more white blood cells.

Conversely, Dr. Kouchakoff's research showed that when people ingested food that hadn't been processed or cooked, their bodies did not respond.

Overcooking foods causes a breakdown in their nutrient value and structure, which either nullifies the benefits they have on our systems, or turns them into substances unrecognizable to the body, which, in turn, elicits an immune response.

To avoid this breakdown, and the breakdown of other foods' nutrient values, all foods should be cooked at a temperature of 200 degrees Fahrenheit or less. This may not always be possible, but according to Dr. Kouchakoff's research, when raw foods were eaten along with cooked foods, the immune response was neutral. So eat raw salad or vegetables along with—not before—cooked meat to ensure that you lessen the potential damage of overcooked foods.

sium, magnesium, manganese, zinc, and copper.

The substance that gives beer its unique bitter taste is called hops, which is credited with delivering a soothing, sedating, and therapeutic effect. In moderate quantities, beer can actually aid your digestive system, help your body transport water, decrease stress, and benefit your heart. There's even new evidence that shows beer can help protect you against cancer.

Oregon State researchers discovered that an antioxidant found in beer may be especially potent.

Antioxidants have been linked to protective effects against atheroscelerosis, cancer, aging, Parkinson's disease, and Alzheimer's disease. Though these findings need to be studied further, it can't hurt to enjoy your frosty mug in the meantime.

And here's even better news. You can forget about the myth that beer makes you fat. Beer is 93 percent water, contains no sugar or fat, and has only low levels of additives. Men with big pot bellies are the minority. And although there is speculation that drinking beer stimulates your appetite, don't let this "infrequent overindulgence" keep you from enjoying it.

If you want more information, there is an excellent website called The Real Beer Page (no affiliation with *The Douglass Report*). You can find it at www.realbeer.com.

Besides containing loads of useful information itself, the site has links to over 150,000 pages of home-brewing splendor and a complete subculture dedicated to brewing and drinking beer.

The truth about salt

Talk about scare tactics—the high-blood-pressure Gestapo is working to convince you that the slightest shake of salt on your food is going to send you to an early grave. They're recommending daily intake quantities that are likely to rob every ounce of flavor from the food you enjoy. Don't stand for it!

Salt, or, more accurately, sodium, is a vital mineral in the human diet. It is the main component of the body's extracellular fluids and carries nutrients to and from cells. Sodium also causes the body to retain water that is needed to perform numerous chemical processes, maintains blood pH, and helps regulate muscle, nerve, and stomach functions. Several studies have proven the benefits of dietary salt.

In the spring of 1995, a report on the results of a four-year study suggested a link between a low-salt diet and higher risk of heart attack. It was published in *Hypertension*, a journal of the American Heart Association.

After studying the effect of sodium on blood pressure in 3,505 subjects, researchers from the University of Toronto suggest that there is a need to reevaluate the entire concept of low-sodium diets. In light of emerging evidence that a low-sodium diet may actually be harmful to some individuals, the researchers said, the objective of universal dietary sodium restrictions should be reevaluated.

The former president of the American Heart Association, Dr. Suzanne Oparil, agrees. Her personal view is that the government may have been too quick to recommend that everyone cut back. "Salt restriction as a solitary recommendation for the population for the prevention or treatment of hypertension is not a powerful weapon and is probably not worth the trouble," she said. According to Oparil, the link between high blood pressure and sodium intake first surfaced about 50 years ago—when studies indicated that hypertension was rare in countries with low salt diets. But salt isn't the only factor in blood pressure levels. So long as you are getting enough calcium, potassium, and magnesium, there's no apparent reason to cut back on salt unless, of course, you just don't like it.

Today, some researchers believe that low-salt diets may actually be dangerous. One theory holds that people with high blood pressure are at greater risk for heart attacks if their kidneys produce excess levels of the enzyme renin.

A low-salt diet causes renin levels to increase. Expect the experts to be duking this out for years to come.

The only salt worthy of your consideration is sea salt from a clean seabed. Don't be fooled: If the label says "U.S. crude salt" it doesn't mean the contents are pure. Crude salt is unrefined industrial salt. It may be unrefined, but it has been mined from a source that is most likely heavily contaminated with heavy metals. Sea salt is the only option. To be a sea salt worthy of your family, it must meet all three of the following criteria:

1) The salt will not be the snow-white variety you're used to. It should be light gray in color. After sitting for a time, the color at the bottom of the container will be darker. If the salt is crystal white, it may be sea salt, but it has been treated and fractionated to rid it of impurities and, at the same time, this rids it of essential minerals. If it is not light gray, it is not a nutritious salt.

2) Legitimate sea salt is not dry to the touch. It should be a little soggy. The moistness is due to the presence of magnesium salts. When kept in cool storage, it doesn't dry out.

3) The crystals, under magnification, are small and cubic. Finding pure sea salt can be rather difficult. There are plenty of products out there claiming to be "pure" but, unfortunately, they have almost all been tampered with to some degree. I have only been able to find one source that I trust—The Grain and Salt Society in Ashville, North Carolina. They can be reached at (800) 867-7258 or on the Internet at www.celtic-seasalt.com.

The healing power of hot peppers

Even if you don't like fiery-hot foods, you should spice up your diet with some chilies.

Capsaicin, the extract that is the main ingredient in the hottest hot sauces on the shelves today, is so full of good stuff it's no wonder someone bottled it.

Capsaicin is an antioxidant and an anti-inflammatory, chockfull of vitamins and beta-carotene. Hot peppers contain calcium, phosphorus, iron, potassium, thiamine (B1), riboflavin (B2), and niacin (B3). They contain more vitamin C than oranges, and they lose only about a third of that after cooking.

In 1982, a study found that chilies thin the blood and lower blood pressure. They also lower the blood level of low-density lipoprotein cholesterol (LDL), the cause of arteriosclerosis. And unlike so many anti-cholesterol agents, they act on the bad cholesterol without affecting the good variety (HDL).

Better yet, a 1986 study published by the American Institute of Nutrition demonstrated that capsaicin reduces the amount of stored fat (triglycerides) in blood cells and reduces blood triglyceride levels.

Chapter 22:

Eat All the Fried Food You Want Without Feeling Guilty or Increasing Your Heart Attack Risk

As they used to say in WWII, "loose lips sink ships." How can I put it in comparison to the misleading headlines we're bombarded with these days? How about, "Loose labels create fables?"

Here's a classic example of how headlines— intentionally or not—shape opinions: "Fried Fish Raises Stroke Risk, Broiled or Baked Reduces it, Study Finds." This was not the correct message, as I will explain.

Here's the way it works: The reader reads the headline: "Fried Fish Raises Stroke Risk." Hmm, he muses, that's interesting. So he reads the first paragraph: "Harvard researchers found in a study of more than 4,700 older people that eating fried fish or fish sandwiches was associated with a higher risk of stroke."

The reader is now completely flummoxed and badly misled. The he goes on to read the details of the article: "...consumption of fried fish or fish sandwiches was associated with a 37 percent higher risk of all kinds of stroke, and a 44 percent higher risk of ischemic stroke, the kind that occurs when a clot blocks an artery." That should end your love affair with fried foods, but it probably won't. And it doesn't necessarily have to.

If you ask most doctors whether fried foods are unhealthy, they would probably say yes. Everyone hears the word "fried" and envisions grease pouring into the liver, the gallbladder groaning in complaint, and the bowels in a discontented and spastic upheaval. Of course, no one knows <u>why</u> fried food is bad. Everybody just knows it is. And while doctors feel confident that they are on sound ground in making the assertion that fried food is probably bad, most of them eat fried foods just like everybody else.

Why you should start at the end

By the time you get to the end of the article the truth about the study finally starts to emerge.

"Another dietary study in the same issue of the journal found the type of fats consumed by middle-aged men might be more important than overall fat intake in reducing the risk of death from cardiovascular disease."

Finally, albeit in a "by-the-way" fashion, they tell readers that it's the <u>type</u> of oil that is important, not the method of cooking.

But that's far from the impression one gets

from the article's headline. And you know as well as I do how short most people's attention spans are (in fact, if you're still reading this, congratulate yourself). Most people will read that ("fried food bad") and think "OK, I knew that—don't need to read the article."

All these people only have half the story and will end up either denying themselves something they really don't have to or feeling guilty about eating things they "know" they shouldn't.

Actions to take:

(1) You can save yourself a lot of hassle—and flavor—knowing the truth about frying. As long as you're using the right kinds of oil (olive, palm, coconut), go ahead and fry away.

(2) When in doubt, eat sushi.

Chapter 23:

Low Fat Dieters Have Higher Heart Risk

It's the biggest nag in modern medicine—one you've heard countless times from mainstream doctors, government health officials, and know-it-all TV talking heads.

Saturated fat is bad for you!

Just one problem with that advice: Saturated fat ISN'T bad for you. In fact, it's absolutely critical to your body and especially to your heart—but don't take my word for it.

Ask the heart patients who took part in a study where half of them were forced to slash their intake of supposedly unhealthy saturated animal fats and increase their intake of supposedly healthy polyunsaturated fats such as safflower oil.

Well... you can try to ask them. Just don't expect too many answers—because the ones who made that switch started dropping like flies.

They died off at DOUBLE the rate of the heart patients who were allowed to keep eating saturated animal fats. They had a higher risk of death from all causes, and more specifically a higher risk of death from heart disease and other heart problems, according to the study in *BMJ*.

What'd I tell you?

Of course, I've been saying this for decades now, and the science has backed me up time and time again. Yet mainstream talking heads and government officials keep telling you to eat your vegetables until you start to sprout yourself.

Then they have the audacity to wonder why heart disease remains our leading cause of death, year after year after year!

Well, it's time to stop the wondering. If you want to protect your heart and live a long and healthy life, eat real butter, real steak, and all the fresh natural animal fats—SATURATED fats—you can handle.

Skip the sugars, skip the carbs, skip the processed foods, and skip the vegetable oils in all their forms.

And if you want to nibble on a plant or two, be my guest—but do it because you want to, not because you have to.

Chapter 24:

Do Vegetarians Live Longer Than Meat Eaters? A New Study Says, "Yes." But the Numbers Don't Add Up

---

You have to ask yourself: Do vegetarians really live longer?

Or do their lives just seem to drag on and on because they never get to indulge in a delicious bacon cheeseburger?

Of course, when a recent vegetarian study was released claiming they outlive us carnivores, the media couldn't jump on it fast enough.

But when you read past the headlines (far past them), you'll see that it's pure farm-raised malarkey!

The "vegetarians-live-longer" study has two low numbers that add up to two huge negatives that the mainstream media completely ignored...

1) The study lasted less than six years.

Six years. Seriously! You cannot gauge longevity in just six years. It's absurd.

If you look at other longevity studies, you'll find a common factor. They're measured in decades. That's "decades"—plural. Maybe the most famous of these studies—The Longevity Project—was started in 1921. And it's still going. THAT'S how you study longevity. It should at least be longer than Seinfeld's run.

2) Ages of subjects ranged from 30 and up.

Ummm... do I really need to point this one out? You can't gauge longevity if part of your cohort hasn't even hit 40 by the time the study is finished. Not even in a third-world country!

But even if this were a 30-year study that started with middle-aged subjects, there would still be one huge problem. Researchers ignored the most important detail about meat eating... The quality of the meat.

Someone who eats high-quality beef from healthy animals that graze on grass is one type of meat eater. Their diet is worlds different from someone who eats sausage, hot dogs, lunch meat, fried chicken, etc. A diet like that is more about highly processed foods than it is about meat.

And it's that second diet that will shorten a lifespan—whether you're eating pork rinds or good old-fashioned, vegetarian French fries.

And contrary to what mainstream nutritionists tell you, good-quality meat contains essential nutrition. And the fat in a first class cut of grass-fed beef is perfect for helping your body absorb fat-soluble vitamins like D, E, and K.

If you choose vegetarianism for religious or ethical reasons, that's one thing. But there is no evidence that a healthy meat-based diet does anything to hurt your longevity—and it will probably make your long life a lot more delicious.

Chapter 25:

RAW DEAL! How Fresh Milk Became a Criminal Enterprise

I can't think of any right more basic than the right to feed your family as you see fit.

Yet that right—that **BASIC** right—is coming under assault by intrusive government bureaucrats who are no longer happy just nagging you about what you "should" eat and drink.

No, these days, they're going further. If nagging won't get you to obey, they'll force you into compliance by passing Nanny State laws against everything from salt to fat to large sodas.

The front line in this war on your freedom to EAT is the battle over raw milk—real, farm-fresh, unpasteurized, unprocessed milk. And this battle is coming to a head around the country, right now, as you read this.

- In Minnesota, a farmer acquitted by a jury of trumped-up charges over raw milk in one county is now fighting those same charges in a neighboring county. So much for the Fifth Amendment!

- In California, a raw milk producer is su-
  ing the FDA, trying to force the agency
  to rule one way or another on the sale
  of milk across state lines in cases where
  it's legal in both states. They tried
  filing a petition first, since the FDA is
  supposed to respond within 180 days—but
  that was FOUR YEARS ago. Good thing jobs
  aren't on the line here. Oh, wait... jobs
  ARE on the line here.

- In Wisconsin, a farmer taking the government to court says he has the RIGHT to
  not only produce raw milk, but—as someone raised in the Amish faith—he has a
  RELIGIOUS OBLIGATION to share his food.
  You can wear a burqa on your drivers' li-
  cense and get away with it in the name of
  religious freedom... but don't you dare
  try to share a little milk!

That's just a small sample of what's going
on at this very moment. In the recent past,
we've also seen **ARMED RAIDS** against ordinary
dairy farmers.

It's an orchestrated campaign of harassment
against the producers, sellers and even consumers of a food product that's been a safe
part of the human diet for some 10,000 years.

Yet despite this long history of safe human
consumption, the feds claim raw milk is suddenly too dangerous to drink—so dangerous it
needs to be restricted and regulated in ways

that not even booze and tobacco are restricted and regulated.

And just like they're lying to you about booze and tobacco, they're lying to you about milk—because their own numbers prove this is one of the safest things you could put into your body.

The feds say there are 10 million drinkers of raw milk in the United States. That's just what they'll admit to—the real numbers are almost certainly higher—but let's use their numbers.

Let's also use their almost certainly exaggerated numbers on illnesses, which link raw milk "outbreaks" to anywhere from a few dozen people to a hundred or so in any given year. It adds up to an illness rate of roughly a thousandth of a percent, give or take, depending on the year.

Meanwhile, everything else—all the foods the feds claim are safe, including "fresh" produce from the big agricultural producers— poison 75 million Americans, or 25 percent of the nation, every single year.

You see where this is going, right?

My friends at the Weston A. Price Foundation crunched the government's numbers recently and found that you're actually ***35,000 times more likely to get sick off foods other than raw milk***. So it's clearly not about safety. If it was, the feds should be urging everyone to drink this stuff.

No, this is really about protecting corporate profits (of course). Ten million consumers drinking raw milk means 10 million fewer people buying Big Dairy's pasteurized (not to mentioned subsidized) supermarket swill.

But no matter how much they try to force little milk producers out of business...no matter how much they threaten, harass, and cajole dairy farmers and milk drinkers alike... no matter how often or how loud they repeat their lies about raw milk... the number of milk drinkers continues to grow.

Drop for drop, there's not a drink on the planet that delivers a bigger health boost. Raw milk is loaded with essential nutrients like calcium, vitamin D, and a natural antibiotic called lactoferrin.

Farm-fresh raw milk is nature's original superfood, and it can help improve digestion, fight asthma and allergies, boost the immune system, aid weight loss, beat pain, and may even help cure autism in children. And that's just the short list.

If you want to know more—if you want the REAL story about REAL milk—get a copy of my book, "The Raw Truth About Milk." You can order it from your local bookshop or online on my website at douglassreport.com (just click on the words "The Raw Truth").

But don't just read about raw milk—be sure to drink it, too. It's worth the extra effort.

Chapter 26:

Pork: Your One-Stop Source for Daily Vegetable Intake...

I recently got an email from someone in Idaho who asked, "Should I cut down on meat and eat more fruits and vegetables?" This person didn't sign his (or her) name, but ladies and gentlemen, I think it's a safe bet to say that we have a newbie on our hands. Anyone who's been reading me for more than a month would be able to answer that question in just one word: Of course not!

But that's okay—we all had to start somewhere. So let's take a step back and look at the big picture. What does a cow eat? Grass, hay, and corn. And what are these? Vegetables. So a steak is nothing more than an efficient mechanism for delivering vegetables to your system. Need grain? Eat chicken. Beef is also a good source of field grass (a green leafy vegetable). And a pork chop can give you 100 percent of your recommended daily allowance of vegetable products.

So, to answer your question, you can cut your fruit and vegetable intake down to ZERO. Eat them if you enjoy them, but not because they're essential to your diet—and certainly not because you think you're saving the life of a furry little creature.

Quite the opposite, in fact. The harvesting of vegetables grown to keep vegetarians (barely) alive takes the lives of millions of small animals daily. Think about it: You won't find a bumper sticker on the back of a combine that says "I brake for small animals." No, those weapons of mass destruction... I mean production... take down everything in their paths—corn, cabbage, carrots, rabbits, foxes, prairie dogs, squirrels, young deer—you name it. So much for the animal rights those veg heads picket for.

Chapter 27:

The Most Disgusting Thing You Could Ever Drink

If you have a weak stomach you might want to brace yourself before you read further. Because if you're drinking plain old tap water, you may as well be drinking from your toilet—AFTER everyone in your neighborhood has used it.

Gross? Yes—but it's true, as a new study confirms that your water is crawling with fecal filth and other nasty stomach-churning germs... and it's getting so bad that bacteria in tap water are now responsible for a fifth of all stomach illnesses in the United States.

That's 1.1 million cases of the squirts, pukes, and worse every single year, according to a new study.

It's like getting Montezuma's Revenge, but without the vacation to Mexico (on the other hand, at least no one's shooting at you when you go to the kitchen sink).

Think better water treatment will help? Think again—your water is already so over-treated that you can probably smell and even taste the bleach and all the other harsh chemicals used to keep it "clean."

Even powerful UV light filters at water treatment plants won't make a difference. After two years of experiments with these systems at water treatment facilities in 14 communities, there was no difference in bacteria levels flowing from faucets in nearby homes, according to the new study.

And there's a simple reason for that: **The bacteria are getting into the water supply AFTER it leaves treatment facilities**.

How does it happen? Join me now as I take you on a journey...

From the toilet to the sink

Try to picture what happens after you flush the toilet. Better yet, don't picture it—it's disgusting. Let's keep it as clean as we can here and say that everything leaves your house in a pipe.

Now, picture what happens when you turn the tap on your sink when you want a drink. Water flows into your home from pipes, right?

They're not the same pipes, of course. But the geniuses who designed these systems generations ago laid both the water and sewer pipes side-by-side in most places.

Must've seemed like a good idea at the time, when the pipes were new and solid and everyone thought they'd last forever, or at least would be replaced from time to time.

But they didn't last, and they haven't been replaced. They're in such bad shape that the EPA says those pipes need $500 billion in repairs and maintenance before the decade's out.

That's HALF A TRILLION BUCKS at a time when our national slush fund is all dried up—so guess what's not getting repaired anytime soon?

That's right... those pipes.

So what you have buried outside your home right now is a crumbling old sewer pipe leaking germs into the soil around it. Running right alongside it, sharing that same dirty soil, is the crumbling old pipe that carries water to your sink—and all it takes is one little crack or leaky spot for the bacteria in the soil to hop inside.

And if there's even a slight pressure change inside the pipes, those germs could actually get SUCKED inside and be given an express ride right to your kitchen sink.

This isn't a theoretical problem. It's a very real one. George Washington University says 850 billion—BILLION, with a "B"—gallons of wastewater enter the drinking water supply every year.

That's more than 100 times the amount of bottled water sold in this country annually.

This is going to get worse, not better.

That's reality—and even if they managed to plug every leak in your pipes or kill off all the bacteria, the water would still be dangerously contaminated with everything from rocket fuel to sex-change hormones.

In fact, in some parts of the country, the water is so overflowing with hormones that fish and frogs are spontaneously changing gender. And if you don't think hormone-laced water has the same effect on humans, check out MTV one of these days.

Yes, it's that bad.

But you don't have to suffer stomach pains or risk a spontaneous sex change—and you certainly don't have to watch your hard-earned cash go down the drain by buying bottled water, either. All you really need is a reverse osmosis filtration system, which you can get right now online or at your local home improvement store.

Reverse osmosis is the only water filtration system that can keep absolutely everything— bugs and drugs—out of your water. Just make sure it's installed where the water enters your home so every tap is protected.

Chapter 28:

New Research Shows Age-Related Blindness Can Be Prevented— With Food

---

Research on how various foods affect health and disease is a tenuous business plagued with many variables, prejudices, and unknowns. Eye health is no exception. However, the latest study on age-related maculopathy (ARM) is worth reporting for a couple of reasons: First and foremost, no one wants to go blind, so any information on preventing the loss of eyesight is noteworthy. But even more important are the study's dramatic results. Researchers found that people who ate just one serving of fish per week drastically cut their risk of blindness.

Age-related maculopathy (ARM) is the leading cause of blindness in the United States. The macula of the eye is where the center of sight is located. The images come through the lens and are focused on the retina, the inner surface of your eye. The macula is the small area on the retina that receives the most light and has the neurological and vascular equipment to handle the load—it's your personal cable modem.

The images are transmitted to the brain through the optic nerve, translated, and then recognized by your brain.

Cut your risk of blindness in half

The "Blue Mountain Eye Study" focused on vision and eye disease among the individuals of an urban population. Food frequency questionnaires were completed by 88 percent of the participants and were used to assess dietary fat and fish intake. The objective of the study was to assess whether dietary intake of fat or fish is associated with the occurrence of ARM.

The retina contains large amounts of polyunsaturated omega-3 fatty acids, specifically docosahexanoic acid (DHA). These fatty acids are necessary for the retina to function normally. Certain types of fish, especially salmon and tuna, also contain large amounts of polyunsaturated omega-3 fatty acids, so the idea is that increasing your consumption of these fish will boost the levels in your retinas, thus protecting your vision.

Fish and vision protection: Less is more

The researchers concluded that increased consumption of fish appeared to protect against late ARM. (Unfortunately, no benefits were associated with fish consumption and the prevention of early stages of ARM.) Those who consumed fish one to three times per month had approximately half the risk of late stage diseases as those who consumed fish less than once per month. The greatest protection was found in those who ate fish once or twice a week. Eating fish more than once or twice a week did not offer any additional benefits.

Actions to take:

Eat fish twice weekly. Salmon, tuna, lake trout, anchovies, halibut, and bass are all readily available in grocery stores and fish markets and have significant amounts of omega-3 fatty acids.

Chapter 29:

It's Not Just How Much You Eat— It's What You Eat. The Real Secret to Diet Success... All Calories Are Not Created Equal!

It's not exactly rocket science: You can lose weight on ANY diet if you just eat less than what your body burns each day.

But just because you can lose weight on the cabbage, vinegar, or Twinkie diet doesn't mean the diet's actually good for you.

And if there's anything worse for your body than a bad diet, it's a gym membership. Exercise can cause injury, joint damage, heart attack, and more—not to mention drain your bank account, too.

For what? For nothing!

The dirty secret of the gym industry is that exercise alone doesn't lead to weight loss. It's been proven time and again that most people simply consume more calories later in the day to compensate for what they burned off in the gym.

Heck, plenty of people don't even wait for "later"—the get all those calories back and then some minutes after the workout, when they suck down a sugar-filled "sports drink."

And then they wonder why they never seem to lose any weight!

Well, forget all that. I'm here to tell you there's a better way—a way to lose weight and **BURN CALORIES** without a bad fad diet and without lifting anything heavier than a forkful of rib eye.

I know that sounds too good to be true, but it IS true: The latest research proves that going low carb will actually cause your body to burn as many extra calories each day as you would punishing yourself in the gym.

Researchers assigned 21 formerly obese patients who had just lost up to 15 percent of body weight to either a low-fat, low-carb, or an in-between diet for a month. Everyone got the same number of calories each day no matter which diet they were put on...but the effects on the body weren't the same at all.

They were completely different.

In fact, the low-carb dieters burned 350 more calories a day than those who went on the low-fat, high-carb diet.

That's the equivalent of a full hour in the gym each day, minus the monthly fee, sweat, and knee pain. In other words, a low-carb diet

has _all the benefits of exercise... without the
actual exercise_!

Those on a "halfway" diet of 40 percent carbs
burned 150 more calories than the folks in the
low-fat, high-carb group. But why go halfway
when you can have the whole hog? Just be sure
to toss the dinner rolls and potatoes (but eat
the skin), and you'll be on your way faster than
you can say "medium rare."

That alone should be enough to get you started—but those aren't all the benefits. Not by
a long shot. The low-carb dieters in the new
study also had better insulin sensitivity, which
means they slashed their risk of diabetes down
the road.

Those who went low-fat, on the other hand,
were already moving down the path towards insulin resistance—making them more likely to get
the disease (and ultimately die of it) later on.

There's no great mystery behind this. Carbs,
especially sugars, cause your blood sugar levels to spike. Eat carb-heavy meals, like the
ones in the typical low-fat diet, and your levels will keep spiking and plunging.

If you could plot your blood sugar levels on
a graph, it would look like the world's wildest
roller coaster ride—and eventually, your poor
pancreas can't take it anymore.

Next thing you know, you've got a main course
of diabetes with a side of heart disease, and
no amount of time in the gym—and no fad diet

in the world—will undo that damage.

Meanwhile, a low-carb diet is proven to keep blood sugar levels stable and well within the safe zone. And now it's proven to actually burn the same number of calories as a full-on gym workout.

All that... and bacon, too. What are you waiting for?

Chapter 30:

The Newest Scam in the Supermarket... Common Foods Are Nothing But Frauds—PROTECT YOURSELF FROM PHONY BALONEY!

It's like the old Folgers Crystals commercials, except instead of secretly replacing your fresh coffee with instant, some companies have done something not nearly so innocent.

They've secretly replaced some of your coffee with something that's not even coffee at all—a cheap filler ingredient, such as worthless ground-up seeds.

And no one is about to jump out with a camera and ask if you can taste the difference. So instead of paying $8 a pound for coffee, you're paying $8 a pound for coffee mixed with seeds—and that's not the only scam going on in your supermarket.

Food fraud is on the rise, with deliberately mislabeled and adulterated foods showing up in nearly every aisle. In the last year alone, there were at least 800 documented new cases of food fraud, according to a report from the U.S.

Pharmacopeial Convention.

Olive oil is mixed with cheap vegetable oils. Expensive pomegranate juice is cut with cheaper ingredients like grape juice—and in at least one case, tests revealed that "100 percent pomegranate juice" didn't contain a drop of actual pomegranate.

Here are a few tricks of the trade you need to watch out for:

SEAFOOD: Low-quality and downright danger-ous fish are deliberately mislabeled and sold to unsuspecting consumers—and it happens **_all the time_**. In many cases, "white tuna" isn't tuna at all, but a dangerous fish called escolar. Escolar is such a major source of food poisoning that it's banned in many nations. Another po-tentially toxic fish, puffer fish, is often sold as monkfish. And high-mercury fish are often con-sistently mislabeled and sold as fish known for low mercury content.

HONEY: Chinese honey is a lot like its toys—contaminated with lead, drugs, and other gar-bage. It's banned in the United States, but "honey laundering" (no, I'm not making this up) strips the honey of all the pollen that would identify its origin. Once stripped of pollen, the honey is sent to a third country such as India before being shipped off to fill plastic bears in the United States. In one survey, 76 percent of supermarket honey was pollen-free—a sure sign of "laundered" Chinese honey.

SPICES: Ground pepper is often mixed with

flavorless ground up seeds. Paprika could be ground up who-knows-what that's been dyed to look like the real thing. And similar tricks are pulled with nearly everything on the spice rack—especially saffron, turmeric, and chili powder.

LEMON JUICE: Fresh lemon juice looks cloudy—but the clouds in bottled juice don't mean it's fresh. Some companies dump chemical phthalates into their lemon juice to give it that cloudy "fresh-squeezed" look. But those phthalates are known endocrine disruptors linked to everything from diabetes and cancer to feminization and low sperm counts. Stick to real lemons, not plastic ones.

That's just a partial list. The USP also found tainted milk, tea, shrimp, cooking oils, and more. If it's sold in a package, you can bet someone is hard at work right now on mixing it with cheap, low-quality, ingredients.

I wish I could tell you there's a surefire way to spot fraud in your food, but there isn't. Obviously, avoid the dollar-store junk and don't trust anything with a "MADE IN CHINA" label.

But even big brands will try to pull the wool over your eyes when they can. Remember that olive oil I mentioned earlier? In a chemical analysis conducted by UC Davis, even top-shelf brands were found to be adulterated with cheaper oils.

The best you can do is shop for fresh ingredients right from the source as much as possi-

ble. And when it's not possible, look for whole
foods. You can hide processed seeds in ground
coffee or pepper. It's a much tougher trick to
pull off with whole beans and peppercorns.

And whatever you buy, do your homework. It
shouldn't be this hard to shop these days, but
it is—so investigate brands and give your money to whoever deserves it, not whoever has the
flashiest labels or the lowest prices.

Chapter 31:

A Cure for Infectious Diseases in a Ray of Light

It's been used to treat asthma, arthritis, AIDS, cancer, and a host of other chronic and terminal diseases. It cured polio in a Los Angeles hospital years before a vaccine was discovered. It has helped physicians in under-funded Russian hospitals successfully treat infectious diseases and major traumas without the use of costly antibiotics. Yet the medical establishment in America today is almost totally ignorant of ultraviolet light therapy... and countless people are suffering—even dying—because of that ignorance.

The theory behind light therapy (also called photoluminescence) is no great secret. We've known for ages that ultraviolet light has antibacterial properties.

It's been used to sterilize medical equipment. At one point, appliance manufacturers even marketed washing machines with built-in ultraviolet light beams.

It was Niels Ryberg Finsen who first demonstrated the healing properties of UV light. In the 1880s, Finsen began providing ultraviolet radiation therapy to patients who had diseases of the skin or mucous membrane. In total, Finsen and his followers treated more than 2,000 people and achieved a success rate of 98 percent. That work earned Finsen the Nobel Prize in 1903.

Subsequent researchers all over the world—from London to Minneapolis—achieved comparable success treating fairly superficial infections, such as mumps, with topical UV light therapy.

Give your immune system an unexpected boost

But in the 1930s, ultraviolet therapy took a giant leap forward. It became a blood treatment. Once again, the theory behind the treatment was quite simple. A physician would draw a sample of blood from a patient, irradiate it with UV light (killing all contagion in the blood cells), and re-inject it into the patient. That cleansing alone would reduce the level of infection inside the patient's body. But something more happened.

In a process that still isn't fully understood today, the irradiation actually strengthened the patient's immune system and helped it eradicate all forms of contagion still in the body, whether they were bacteria or viruses.

In 1944, two researchers from Washington State, Dr. Virgil K. Hancock and Mr. Emmett K. Knott, presented their findings on blood irradiation: "Clinical experiments have further determined [that] the beneficial energy [is] stored up in the rayed blood temporarily, and if such blood can be returned to the bloodstream immediately after it has been irradiated, it will throw off secondary irradiation which will stimulate and energize the patient."

By that point, the two researchers had treated more than 6,500 patients with their ultraviolet blood therapy.

Many of those patients had life-threatening infections and had failed to respond to conventional treatment, namely sulfa drugs. The UV treatment worked in virtually every case, and caused no harmful side effects.

Light therapy: a polio miracle

Around the same time, ultraviolet therapy was working a small miracle in a Los Angeles hospital. Like virtually every other hospital across America at the time, the facility was admitting a steady stream of polio patients. Struggling to breathe, most were deteriorating rapidly and facing little chance of a full recovery, if they survived at all.

Two physicians, George Miley and Jens Christensen, began administering ultraviolet blood irradiation therapy on desperate cases. The results were phenomenal. Of the 58 people they treated, only one died—an 18-year-old girl with advanced bulbar polio (polio of the brain stem which typically kills 40 percent of its victims). Most of the other patients, however, experienced rapid relief of toxic symptoms.

On September 12, 1946, for example, a 7-year-old boy was hospitalized with a temperature of 104 and definite signs that he was suffering from bulbar polio. Doctors told the boy's parents that he had a 1 in 20 chance of surviving. Dr. Miley, however, irradiated 44 cc's of the boy's blood the day he arrived at the hospital. By midnight, the boy's fever disappeared and his pulse and respiration began returning to normal. Two weeks later, he was discharged. Just 3 1/2 months after that, his father reported that "had one not known that the child had had polio, no present sign would suggest it."

In patients with spinal polio—an extremely toxic disease that induces rapid muscle and respiratory deterioration—light therapy dramatically eased symptoms within 48 to 72 hours. Five patients who were considered in imminent danger of dying, recovered after receiving irradiation treatments.

Miley and Christensen even tried the technique on a 23-year-old woman who was on the brink of death and was being sustained on a respirator. She was also 7 months pregnant. The woman began to recover 24 hours after her third irradiation treatment and went on to deliver a normal infant at term—a first for a polio patient in California.

Save money—and lives—
in cash-strapped Russian hospitals

Within a few years, however, the medical pro-

fession largely abandoned light therapy in fa-
vor of newly developed antibiotics. But a few
of us continued to explore the potential of
this treatment.

Human trials in Philadelphia demonstrated
UV's ability to ease severe bronchial asthma. Surgeons discovered that photoluminescence could effectively treat thrombo-phlebitis
(blood clots that constitute one of the most
unpredictable and dangerous complications of
surgery). One report on five patients noted that
pain and tenderness eased rapidly within 24 to
48 hours after treatment (and all the patients
had previously failed to respond to antibiotic
treatment). Even researchers at Yale University
began using UV irradiation of blood to treat
cancer patients.

But the most striking developments in photoluminescence recently have come from an unex-
pected source—Russia.

From what I've seen, medical practice in Russia and other former Soviet-bloc countries has
tended to lag several decades behind Western medicine. So when I visited St. Petersburg in 1991
to investigate the use of light therapy there, I
expected to find a practice in its infancy.

I expected to spend my time enlightening my
backward Eastern colleagues. Was I in for a
surprise!

At St. Petersburg's Pasteur Institute (which
is a government agency, not an affiliate of the
Pasteur Institute in France), scientists have

been pioneering new medical uses for phototherapy for 20 years and passing their findings
along to physicians throughout the country.

Surgeons in Russia have used UV blood irradiation therapy on more than 100,000 patients...
and reduced post-operative complications by 50
percent. By drawing blood from a patient, irra-
diating it, and injecting it back into the patient in a process of autotransfusion, surgeons
have eliminated the patient's risk of developing compatibility problems with donor blood.
Likewise, emergency physicians have successfully used UV therapy on thousands of Russians
suffering from severe trauma or third degree
burns.

For the Russians, light therapy is much more
than a fascinating new medical technique. It's
a way to treat patients without the use of expensive antibiotics. And in a country where
drugs are costly and hospital budgets are mea-
ger, low-cost light therapy can help physicians
heal a lot more patients and end a lot more
suffering.

Action to Take:

*Unfortunately, Americans have limited access
to photoluminescence.*

*I have wrestled with this dilemma for years.
The obstacles are multiple: ignorant, un-
interested, or antagonistic doctors; op-
pressive medical systems at the state and
federal level; and collusion, that borders
on the criminal, between the FDA and the*

drug industry (which, of course, wants to protect its monopoly over treatments).

You are not totally without options, however. Contact the American College for Advancement in Medicine (ACAM) and ask for the names of doctors who use this treatment or who might be willing to try it. Call them at (800)532-3688 or go online to www.acam.org.

Chapter 32:

The Rise of the 'MYSTERY' Disease: The Symptoms... The Cause... THE CURE

It's the silent epidemic sweeping the nation—a wave of illness striking from coast to coast.

And the so-called experts haven't even noticed.

They've missed all the usual warning signs because the usual warning signs aren't there. There's no common set of symptoms to watch for... it doesn't spread from person to person... and there are no clusters of sick people to get anyone's attention.

In some cases, it's a physical disease with pain and fatigue. In others, it's a mental condition with moodiness, irritability, or memory loss. What makes this mystery disease so hard to spot is that it's a world-class mimic that can impersonate so many other conditions.

And it does it so well that your doc is bound to diagnose it wrong.

When he gets that diagnosis wrong, you get the wrong treatment. And when you get the wrong treatment, you don't get better.

You get WORSE.

Well, if you've got a few unexplainable symptoms of your own and you're **sick** of seeing doctor after doctor and specialist after specialist... **tired** of coming up empty after so many tests you feel like a human pincushion... **frustrated** with treatments that don't work because they're for diseases you don't even have... then I've got some **good news** for you for a change.

Your own doctor might not have a clue as to what's going on, but I do—and if you take action now, you can reverse this mystery disease and get back to life the way it was before disaster struck.

The reason so many doctors and specialists keep getting this one wrong is because they're all looking in the wrong place. In fact, this mystery "disease" isn't actually a disease at all.

IT'S A POISON!

Mercury is one of the most toxic heavy metals on earth—and odds are, it's slowly building up inside your body right now. It's in your food, your water, and even your teeth.

No wonder you're falling apart!

If you want to see how fast your world can crumble, take a look at the case of Richard Gelfond. You may not know his name, but you've heard of his company. Gelfond is CEO of IMAX, the movie theater chain known for its giant screens.

Once upon a time, Gelfond was vibrant and athletic. Then, out of the blue, he found himself getting weaker and weaker. It reached the point where he needed to cling to his wife to cross the street.

Gelfond recently told "60 Minutes" that doctors on both coasts couldn't figure out why he was rapidly deteriorating. Then, a neurologist asked him about his diet.

Turns out he was eating seafood twice a day—a habit that nearly cost him his life, because the fish he was eating had more mercury lurking in it than an old thermometer.

He's undergoing treatment now, but tragically it may be too late: While he's improved, Gelfond says his life might never be the same again. And if a man with all that money and access to top doctors can't get the help he needs in time, what chance do you as a "Regular Joe" have?

Well, your chances suddenly got much better just now... because unlike Richard Gelfond, you have ME to keep watch over you.

The first thing you need to do, whether you have any signs of mystery disease or not, is to identify and eliminate all the possible sources of mercury exposure.

Odds are, you've got more than you think.

Seafood: Love fish? Then, like Gelfond, you probably already have elevated mercury levels. In one recent study, 84 percent of fish sampled tested positive for mercury. High-mercury fish include tuna, shark, and king mackerel, but the truth is almost any fish can be contaminated these days. Choose wisely.

Teeth: If you have a mouthful of silver fillings, you've got a mouthful of mercury—and you weren't just exposed when the dentist did the job. Over the years, the fillings slowly crumble—and you get a dose of mercury with every bite, chew, and swallow. The dentists of the International Academy of Oral Medicine and Toxicology specialize in mercury-free dentistry and the safe removal of amalgam ("silver") fillings. Visit them online at iaomt.org to find a dentist near you.

Light bulbs: If mercury in your mouth is the worst idea ever, then a cloud of hot mercury suspended in a thin glass tube a few feet above your head for 12 hours a day has got to be a close runner-up. Yet that's exactly what the federally mandated "environmentally friendly" CFL light bulbs are. I'm no fan of the old bulbs, but stock up while you still can—or make the switch to full-spectrum lighting.

Water: Yes, there's even mercury in your tap water, often a byproduct of industrial waste and the chemicals used on factory farms. Amazingly, the feds didn't even start regulating mercury in the water until the 1990s—so many of us have been drinking, cooking with, and bathing in contaminated H20 for decades. Don't count on your local water department to keep the mercury out. They don't even know where to begin. A reverse osmosis water filter can remove up to 97 percent of the mercury.

There's also mercury in everything from vaccines to skin creams—supposedly just a "little bit" here and there. But when it comes to this toxic heavy metal, every little bit counts—because once it enters your body, it doesn't leave.

It stays, slowly accumulating with each exposure. It may take years or even decades before you reach toxic levels, but when you do... WHAM! You've got "mystery disease."

Like I said earlier, the symptoms can be physical, mental or both—which is why it's so often misdiagnosed. Here are just **some** of the common conditions that could really be mercury poisoning in disguise:

- Parkinson's disease
- Cerebral palsy
- Tremors
- Respiratory problems
- Hearing loss
- Alzheimer's disease
- Sleep disorders
- Fatigue
- Headaches
- Muscle pain and weakness
- Pain
- Multiple Sclerosis
- Fibromyalgia
- Stomach disorders
- Vision loss
- Skin diseases
- Dementia
- Depression
- Irritability
- Mood swings
- Metabolic encephalopathy
- And more!

Some people will have only one of those symptoms. Others may have several. And still others could experience something else entirely—so you can see what even a good doctor is up against here.

Testing for mercury isn't difficult. But it's not routine, and it does take a certain amount of work. Because there are different types of mercury (leading to different symptoms), there are different tests—and a good doctor will use more than one, including a blood test, 24-hour urine collection, fecal tests, skin tests, and an analysis of your hair.

If you suspect mercury poisoning and one test comes back negative, insist on taking some of the other tests.

If mercury poisoning is detected, early treatment is critical. In many cases, chelation therapy can help remove some forms of mercury.

A naturopathic physician can help diagnose you and choose the best treatment. I recommend a doctor who belongs to the American Academy for Advancement in Medicine. To find one near you, call 1-800-532-3688 or visit them online at acam.org.

Chapter 33:

The Worst Condition You Don't Know You Have—And the Best Way to Make It Go Away Fast

---

As soon as I tell you what this article is about, a lot of you will be tempted to stop reading. Don't. That could be a most dire mistake, one that virtually guarantees that many of the symptoms you're experiencing are here to stay.

You see, there is a highly aggressive, opportunistic pathogen that attaches to everyone, literally everyone has it. And when it starts to take over, as it so often does, it can cause such a wide list of symptoms (more than 100!)— from migraines to irritable bowel to memory loss—that most doctors don't connect them.

In fact, if you mention this single cause to most mainstream doctors, they will probably deny it, dismiss it, and disagree. And that can keep you sick for a very long time.

But not if you keep reading.

The information you're about to read will

change your life. All those nagging "incurable" symptoms you've been plagued with... they'll disappear. And you'll remember what it feels like to feel good, really good. All it takes is one proven treatment, just a few sips a day. Problems solved.

The hidden dangers of these insidious microbes... and what you can do about them

If you've been suffering from what seems like an unending stream of mysterious symptoms and illnesses, be prepared to take action to make it all stop. Because there's a better than good chance that a lot of what's ailing you stems from a single insidious cause, one with an enormous influence on almost every aspect of your health.

It's a tiny microbe, *candida albicans*, better known as yeast (but this is not just about yeast infections). It occurs naturally in and on your body, and everybody has it. Candida lives mainly in your large intestine, where it doesn't do much harm...until things get out of control.

When you're healthy, your body hosts enough beneficial bacteria to keep that yeast in check, and they seem to coexist in harmony. But when your good bacteria get depleted, sadly a very common occurrence, candida can get the upper hand. And it doesn't take much to let that happen:

- Antibiotics
- Steroids

- Poor diet
- High blood sugar

- Hormonal changes
- Stress
- Heavy metal toxicity
- Chemotherapy and radiation

When the candida overgrowth is severe enough to take control, your health can quickly go from bad to worse. And at its worst, systemic candidiasis, the effects can be very dangerous.

Even in less severe cases, your body will become rundown and exhausted as your immune system desperately tries to fight off the invasion. And that can make you even more vulnerable to other infections.

So proper treatment is crucial, but it can be hard to find.

The only way to win is to fight the right enemy

There are conventional pharmaceutical treatments for candida—and they can work, to a point. Many doctors won't write (and most insurance companies won't cover) prescriptions for candida other than a typical yeast or skin infection. And these drugs are designed for short-term use, not really for chronic conditions, so taking them long-term can pose a whole new set of threats to your system.

Natural solutions can be helpful, too, but even they can have a hard time overcoming candida that's gone out of control.

Because there's a growing problem that's difficult to address.

There are now more than 63 forms of candida.

Many of them have appeared recently, thanks to GMO crops and bioengineering. And they can be very hard to control. Plus, different strains of candida produce different symptom patterns, effecting different body systems. Add to that this microbe's ability to cause a broad spectrum of elusive symptoms... and you begin to see the problem.

The solution comes in a powerful candida cocktail

Dr. Frank King has practiced holistic health care for decades, and he's been instrumental in creating a hugely successful fast-working candida elimination formula. And thanks to this proprietary homeopathic candida cocktail, you can wipe out your candida overgrowth, and let

---

Think your symptoms are unrelated? Think again

Telltale symptoms of the insidious invader cover a wide range of issues, and most people—most doctors—never see the connection. Here's a tiny sample of what you could be facing.

- ❑ Impotence
- ❑ Trouble concentrating
- ❑ Athlete's foot
- ❑ Vaginitis
- ❑ Itchy ears
- ❑ Bladder infections
- ❑ Nasal congestion
- ❑ Dizziness
- ❑ Wheezing
- ❑ Rapid heartbeat
- ❑ Constipation
- ❑ Diarrhea
- ❑ Mood swings
- ❑ Chest pain
- ❑ Abdominal bloating
- ❑ Sugar cravings
- ❑ Irritability
- ❑ Heartburn
- ❑ Aversion to strong smells
- ❑ Chemical sensitivities
- ❑ Adult acne
- ❑ Eczema
- ❑ Stomach pain
- ❑ Muscle aches
- ❑ Joint pain
- ❑ Frequent headaches
- ❑ Chronic fatigue

your body's beneficial bacteria flourish again.

The formula is so important because "candida is a factor in 80 percent of chronic disease patients," he told me. "And since everyone has some candida, it's elusive to measure and diagnose, especially when the symptoms can seem so unrelated."

AquaFlora High Potency 9 (HP9), so-named because it originally covered nine candida strains, first came to be in 1990. Since then, Dr. King's company (KingBio) has tweaked the formula to broaden that candida cocktail as new strains have been discovered.

And along with that multi-strain mix, the formula contains 22 supportive homeopathic ingredients and three botanicals. The homeopathic ingredients will help relieve symptoms very quickly, sometimes beginning even with the first dose. The flower essences are there to offer emotional support—because candida can impact and imbalance your sense of wellbeing.

Strengthen your body to keep candida overgrowth from coming back

Candida has a well-deserved bad reputation. It's tough, resistant, hard to clear, and itching to take over.

And depending on which strains you have, and how long they're around, they can begin to destroy the integrity of your GI tract. Candida dominates, and takes the place of good, essential bacteria, leaving your GI system and your immune system (70 percent of that is in your GI tract) at risk.

Over time, this can damage your intestines, and lead to conditions like leaky gut and irritable bowel syndrome, making it ever harder to regain a healthy bacteria balance.

But AquaFlora HP9 gives you the edge over candida, no matter what strain has taken hold. And the gentle homeopathic approach seems to help most people avoid troubling candida "die-off" reactions (see the sidebar).

Rather, most people start to feel better right away.

"There's not one person who doesn't need this product"

Dr. Deanna Karson, chiropractor, has seen incredible changes in her patients' lives...and her own... ever since she brought AquaFlora HP9 into her practice.

Though she didn't have a classic yeast infection, she suspected candida might be the culprit

---

If this is working, why do I feel worse?

If you've got a serious yeast overgrowth, you may experience some initial discomfort as the candida starts to die off. This is formally known as a Herxheimer reaction.

As the yeast dies, it can give off toxins. When a lot of yeast dies off, that's a lot of toxins released into your body, which can cause some temporary side effects (like diarrhea). But once those toxins are flushed out of your system (usually very quickly), you'll begin to feel much better.

for her bloated stomach and sugar cravings. She knew her "guts were fighting something." So she tried HP9 to see what would happen.

Within one week, her stomach "went flat—it seemed like it had shaved off the bloating and distension I had before." Now, Dr. Karson still takes a maintenance dose (she's on her third bottle) to keep those very uncomfortable symptoms from creeping back. And based on her personal success story, she recommends AquaFlora HP9 to the overwhelming majority of her patients.

"Nine out of ten of my patients take it, even the men. And they've seen huge improvements in so many areas:

- Clear thinking

- Better bowel movements

- Gas, bloating, and distension are all gone

- Pain throughout the body eases up

- Headaches get minimized, or disappear

- Itching and rashes clear up

On top of that, almost everyone loses weight, up to 45 pounds! The smallest loss I've seen was ten pounds."

When I asked Dr. Karson about side effects and Herxheimer reactions, she told me she'd seen it in three patients, all of whom had undergone radiation treatment for cancer. The symptoms tapered off within a couple of weeks as all the toxins left their bodies, but it was rough going at first. "People who've been on chemotherapy or radiation, or have toxic heavy metal exposure, may get bigger reactions as the toxins clear."

Still, she believes High Potency 9 is appropriate for everyone. "There's not one person who doesn't need this product," she told me. "When you get your GI tract clean and maintain that, your body can fight harder and stay healthier."

Take AquaFlora High Potency 9™ to conquer candida completely

AquaFlora High Potency 9 is your first-line solution to conquer candida overgrowth and free yourself from all the symptoms it can cause.

The manufacturer recommends taking one capful, twice daily. Doses should be taken on an empty stomach, before breakfast and at bedtime. Most people notice some symptom relief almost immediately, but for some it may take a few days.

If you've had candida for a long time, you might want to try additional AquaFlora homeopathic support products to help your body heal completely.

The candida-sugar connection

Did you ever have a sugar craving? Well, it might not be you craving for that cookie after all—it might be the candida. Yeast absolutely requires sugar to survive, so it triggers intense cravings, practically forcing you to eat sweets. But get rid of the candida, and you might get rid of that sweet tooth along with it.

Enzyme Restoration™ helps relieve upper GI symptoms (like heartburn, nausea, and lactose intolerance) and aid healthy digestion.

Probiotic Restoration™ offers lower GI restoration and support, relieving lower GI symptoms like cramps, abdominal swelling, diarrhea, and constipation. It also helps your body restore and maintain beneficial bacteria.

Heavy Metal Detox™ helps address the oddly very common candida-heavy metal connection. This formula relieves symptoms such as fatigue, headaches, twitching muscles, and unhealthy skin.

You can find ordering information for Aqua-Flora High Potency 9™ and its homeopathic support products in your Wellness Directory on page 409.

Chapter 34:

FLU SHOT MADNESS!
Why Doctors Refuse the Shot—
And You Should, Too

If anyone on this planet knows all about the flu and flu shots, it's healthcare workers. They read the studies and talk about them around the water cooler the way most people talk about the football game.

(OK, so healthcare workers talk about the football game, too—but then they talk about the studies.)

More importantly, they treat flu patients every day—and that means they're exposed to the virus every day. Yet doctors, nurses, and other healthcare workers REFUSE the shot in droves.

Think they know something you don't? You bet they do—and I'll let you in on their secret in a moment.

But first, if you're in the healthcare industry yourself, your body is no longer yours. It belongs to the government—because across the nation, healthcare workers are being ordered to get the shot...or get lost.

In Colorado, for example, hospitals have to report flu shot "compliance" levels and start handing out pink slips when they don't reach government-mandated targets.

Don't want a flu shot? Tough!

Worried about the very real risks? Quit whining!

Read a study that shows they don't work? Stop all that reading and roll up your sleeve!

The claim, as always, is that this forced vaccination program is for the "greater good." But I don't see what's so great here—doctors and nurses don't want to be sick with the flu anymore than you do.

And when they refuse the shot, they know exactly what they're doing.

First, they know that **the flu shot isn't safe**. They know that despite the CDC's constant noises to the contrary, the vaccine can actually CAUSE the flu.

For example, five studies out of Canada found that people vaccinated with the 2008-2009 flu shot were actually more likely to come down with swine flu than those who weren't vaccinated—but instead of causing alarm, it was dismissed as "the Canadian problem."

That's right... don't blame the shot. Blame Canada!

But in a new study, ferrets given the shot

were more likely to get swine flu than ferrets given a placebo shot—and since ferrets don't carry passports, you can't dismiss this as a "Canadian problem" after all.

And that's not the only problem—Canadian or otherwise—with flu shots.

The swine flu shot, for example, has been linked to everything from paralyzing nerve disorders to an outbreak of narcolepsy to dozens of deaths. "Normal" flu shots aren't much better, with common side effects that include fever, fatigue, headaches, muscle pain, and more.

Throw in some sniffles, and it sounds to me like the "side effects" and the flu are pretty much one in the same.

For all those risks, the shot isn't even very effective at preventing the flu. One recent analysis found the absolute reduction in risk is just 1.5 percent, and I think even that's wildly optimistic.

Another major analysis, for example, found the flu shot doesn't reduce the rate of hospitalization and doesn't slow the spread of the disease—and that most of the studies to find any benefit at all were rigged by vaccine makers.

That's the kind of research doctors talk about around the water cooler—and that's why you should make like a healthcare worker yourself if anyone asks you to roll up your own sleeve and just say "NO!"

At least you still have a choice... for now.

Chapter 35:

The "BLOOD SUGAR BOMBSHELL" That Could Change It All!

It can be worse than the sugar "spikes..."

More tiring than the endless hours of exercise they want you to endure...

More gruesome than the bowls of birdseed they want you to eat to stay healthy...

Yeah.

You know what I'm talking about... The **nagging**. After 40 years of marriage, your 'better half' doesn't hold back on anything... from what you're wearing to what you're eating. And you always hear the constant drum of...

"Put that down..."

"You can't have this..."

"You can't have *that*..."

"What are you *thinking*?"

"Are you even listening to me?"

<u>Enough already</u>!

Wouldn't you just love to put a sock in all of those traps?

Today, I'm going to show you a **bold breakthrough that can do it**. With the help of just one, simple step... Become the boss of your blood sugar...And silence the nagging—FOR GOOD!

It's all thanks to what I believe has the potential to be this century's most exciting breakthrough in metabolic science.

In fact... I think it may one day be remembered as... The "BLOOD SUGAR BOMBSHELL" that changed it all.

If you're waiting for the new sugar metabolism miracle that could finally help halt all that harping—get ready... The wait is over.

Now I can't promise to end the nagging about what you're wearing or when you're going to clean out the garage. But I do have a little something extra in my arsenal to keep you healthy and get the food police off your back. Just let me ask you...

How many *demeaning* hand slaps is it going to take?

How many disapproving glares can you possibly handle?

How many "high and mighty" rants are you going to sit through before...

You finally SNAP?

...maybe sooner than you think because I gotta say... It really seems like the health nags are out in full force over blood sugar these days...

Everyone from doctors to grandkids thinks that they're a downright "glucose guru."

Well I want to know... If we have so many experts at our disposal then please tell me— why in the heck are more people struggling with blood sugar concerns than ever?!

You and I both know it... something is broken. It's turning into a downright catastrophe—

But you know what?

You don't have to eat like a bird... Or jog like a fitness freak...

Of course, you can't go raiding a candy store or surfing the day away on the couch... I think we both know a little good ol' fashioned exercise and eating healthy, low-carb, balanced meals are always the best plan. And pushing away from the table before you chomp down that piece of pie wouldn't hurt, either.

But you definitely don't have to be treated like a 2-year-old to keep your blood sugar in check.

The very first step (and the most fun, might I add) is to plug up your ears good and tight... and tune out the noise as best you can, because those "experts" know as much about glucose as I know about winning a beauty pageant.

It's a truth that only a few doctors are waking up to...

And here it is...

There is a COLOSSAL "missing piece" to the blood sugar debate.

The "know-it-all" doctors and all of those health nags want you to think they have it all figured out—but they couldn't be more wrong.

I'll show you why in just one moment, but first... let me explain something.

Let's be candid...

Of course you have to watch your diet—but sometimes... cookies happen. And even that so-called "healthy diet" so many of the nags want you to follow is still filled with carbs, carbs, carbs. What you really need to put a sock in their traps is...

A better way to protect yourself from the nasty effects of sugar spikes, NATURALLY

This is BIG NEWS.

(I just love shutting up the health nags when I can... And I really shut them up this time.)

Look, you've been made to feel like a toddler. Just because you're getting older doesn't mean you have to constantly be watched, scrutinized and judged... You've managed to take care of yourself and stay healthy all your life, and your not going to stop now.

You hear the same old things... over and over... and you still worry about your blood sugar.

It's time you discovered a complete "blood

sugar bombshell" that can help make it so...

This won't just be some dream. It could be your new day.

I gotta say, I'm bouncing off the walls like a kid in a candy factory to show you this break-through because...

I know how much it's going to change your life.

Heck... It's what I expect to be remembered as the "blood sugar bombshell" that changed it all. And you're at the right place, at the right time to get in on the action.

But I'm getting ahead of myself. Before I show you what could be a revolution in how we think about blood sugar support...

I must tell you why I consider this discovery the "Sugar Shot" heard round the world!

This mighty marvel was born because doctors are finally starting to ask the right question—the same question I've been asking for years...

What's so wrong with shoving your pie hole full of pasta and cake all day? Especially if you skip dinner—why can't you just eat a bowl of ice cream instead?

Does that seem like a silly question to you?

Make no mistake, the blood sugar spikes caused by eating too much pasta and potato chips are something to be concerned about, but when you ask a doctor that question, plenty of them will reply with, "they just ARE."

Nope. That's not good enough for me and it shouldn't be acceptable to you.

Because when you do some due diligence and start to analyze the "why," you find something BIG.

When you eat a meal, especially one that's high in carbs and sugar, your blood glucose levels spike and sugar gets pushed into your cells to use for energy. (Carbs are notorious sugar spikers—that's why I've always pushed for more meat, more eggs, and less cake.)

But for decades doctors have been next to clueless about what exactly happens when blood sugar gets into your cells.

But this new understanding in how sugar metabolism works is wiping the medical drawing board clean.

It's something I like to call a "medical mind shift." It's like realizing your 20-step equation isn't working because you screwed up on step one.

But when you look at how sugar is used by your cells with a new set of eyes...

EUREKA! The floodgates bust wide open and a new breakthrough comes racing down the pipeline.

So what is it?

What has scientists, researchers and doctors racing through U.S. labs with newfound enthusiasm?

What could transform our very understanding

of how our cells manage sugar for the next 100 years and beyond?

Oh yes. It's THAT BIG. And I've been blaring on about this revelation for years...

Animal and *in vitro* studies suggest it could...

- Prevent glucose damage to your cells

- BOOST a "secret enzyme" within your cells that acts like a sugar spike watchdog

- Promote the health of your vision, your skin, your brain, heart and MORE

Don't believe it? You will in a few moments because in reality...it just makes sense.

Most doctors will nag you till you cry *"MERCY!"* But what you really need is more of this secret "watchdog" enzyme.

What you're about to discover is breakthrough science.

It's a bold approach.

But it's also the perfect sense support that may help maintain healthy cells and tissues in contact with glucose.

I have a theory as to why blood sugar health is turning into the next "Worldwide Obsession."

It's because most "know-it-all" doctors are missing a colossal piece to the puzzle.

Take a look...

There is one HUGE reason why...

Modern medicine is Wrong, Wrong, Wrong on blood sugar...

You always hear the same thing...

There are no new natural solutions for maintaining healthy blood sugar metabolism, so work with what we've got—WRONG!

I'm going to show you 3 natural solutions right now.

One is the cutting-edge "sugar spike safeguard" I'm itching to tell you about...

One is so promising that even a current USDA researcher is standing up and singing its praise...

And one sets the standard for all blood sugar supporters, and if yours doesn't have it, you've got a dud.

And when you put them all together—you get the BLOOD SUGAR BOMBSHELL that will change the way we think about natural blood sugar support.

But first... take a look at the "medical mind shift" taking place *right now* and how cellular protection against blood sugar spikes may never be the same again.

It starts with...

The SUGAR SPIKE WATCHDOG that was missing from modern science for decades...

It's called *transketolase* (trans-KEE-toh-lase).

It's the colossal missing piece I'm so excited about because it acts like a dedicated watchdog against the hidden enemy I'll explain in a moment.

You see, your body's natural insulin pushes glucose through cell membranes...

That's all well and good. It's fine, but that's only half the battle. Remember when I asked why bingeing on sugar is such a big deal? It's because of...

The SHOCKING SIDE EFFECT behind each and every sugar spike

When you eat white bread, cookies, pastas or other high glycemic meals—it sends your blood sugar levels sky high and fast.

Of course if you know me, I'd always choose a fat juicy steak for most meals but now and again, sugar sneaks in.

And these spikes are cause for concern because when your cells come in contact with excess blood sugar—a nasty thing happens and *advanced glycation end products* (AGEs) are created.

What the heck are they? AGEs naturally form in everyone's body, even the most health-obsessed fitness nuts and nutrition nuts. But eating sugar and processed foods can cause even more AGEs to form. Why are they so bad? AGEs literally age your body prematurely—important parts, too like your eyes, your skin, your blood vessels and especially your heart.

It's the missing piece to the blood sugar debate. Eating healthy is a critical component in maintaining healthy blood sugar—but sugar spikes WILL happen, and when they do—you have to protect your cells and vital organs from AGEs. And that's exactly what this "watchdog" enzyme, transketolase, does... it helps battle the production of AGE's in the first place—helping to protect your most valuable assets in the process.

But while you can promote your body's healthy insulin response...was there a way to promote your body's transketolase activity?

The hunt was on for...

A smarter, bolder alternative to fight back against sugar spikes!

And *boy, oh boy,* IT HAS BEEN FOUND.

Imagine a secret that can charge this enzyme and *in vitro* and animal studies have shown it may help...

- **Protect you against elevated glucose's reckless activity—helping to... keep your vision sharp, your kidneys healthy and your heart pumping strong**

- **Fight the formation of damaging AGEs...**

- **Finally give you ammunition to help shut up the health nags**

It's time to pull back the curtains so you could fight the damaging effects of sugar spikes.

The breakthrough happened in Japan, but at the time, no one realized what they had discovered...

During the 60's, Japanese researchers were fascinated with a natural substance called **benfotiamine**.

Why? Because it showed promising results in supporting nerve function.

The Japanese researchers made notes of benfotiamine's power... how they thought it worked... and what it was made of...

Heck, it was even patented in 1962... but its true potential was never quite realized. Then it all but disappeared.

For over 40 years, this untapped powerhouse remained underground.

Sure, there would be a mention of "interesting results" in the back pages of a medical journal every now and again...

But in America for the most part, this giant stayed fairly well hidden.

That is, of course, until I got involved.

I first wrote about benfotiamine's incredible potential in the December 2003 issue of my medical newsletter.

In my search to create a complete "blood sugar bombshell"—I caught wind of an animal study taking place with benfotiamine and glucose. The study revealed that benfotiamine has the potential to help provide unheard of protection to cells in contact with glucose.

The more I unearthed about benfotiamine's history, the more I was convinced...

This was the breakthrough I had been looking for

I immediately wrote my article and shouted its praises to anyone who would listen.

Very few would——why?

Maybe it's because this marvel works *too well*. Substances with this kind of potential have a way of keeping profit-hungry bigwigs up at night.

Or maybe it was because it was too rare, too underground and too hard to get your hands on to make any sense.

Or maybe... The mainstream wasn't prepared to admit they overlooked a crucial piece of the blood sugar puzzle.

But to understand why this discovery is so special you have to do something that the mainstream is always reluctant to do...

START FROM SCRATCH.

When you wipe the drawing board bare... When you take a microscope to sugar metabolism——

Seeing where it starts...

The exact chain reaction involved...

And what top-notch protection looks like...

You find something BIG.

There is a critical vitamin involved in sugar metabolism.

It helps your cells fight the formation of AGEs when they come into contact with excess glucose caused by eating the occasional carbo-loaded meal. In fact, it's essential in the formation of the "watchdog" enzyme, transketolase. This remarkable vitamin is called _thiamine_ and...it's very smart.

And you want to know the biggest revelation?

Researchers have discovered that people battling blood sugar concerns often displayed low levels of thiamine...

This is the "missing link" I've been searching for.

But... it's not that simple.

You can judge thiamine's effectiveness by how it boosted the "watchdog" enzyme, transketolase. And standard thiamine only increases this enzyme by a measly 25 percent...

Not exactly the revolution in support you deserve...

The problem is that thiamine is a water-soluble vitamin. Plain and simple—it rushes out of your body too fast to have much of an impact.

If only there was a _fat-soluble_ thiamine that

could stick around in the body to really pack a punch.

Remember those Japanese researchers I told you about? Remember *their* special discovery, benfotiamine? The very same discovery I've been hollering about for 9 years.

Benfotiamine just happens to be a fat-soluble derivative of thiamine...

Not only that, but its unique structure enables it to more easily pass through cell membranes and your body absorbs benfotiamine about 5 times as well as conventional thiamine!

Sounds good in theory, right? But what about results?

One researcher heard of benfotiamine's potential and thought he'd give it a shot.

But what happened next could never have been predicted...

The fat-soluble vitamin, discovered so long ago in Japan...

Increased activity of the "watchdog" enzyme by 250 percent *in vitro*

And guess what?

Combined with the other breakthroughs you're about to discover, it's sure to silence the non-stop nagging.

How? Wait until you see this...

The complete blood sugar bombshell you're

about to discover can help you stay healthy. Stay strong. And stay charged with vim and vigor.

With that extra natural support helping to keep your blood sugar levels healthy, you'll be surprised how much more energy you could have.

You'll shine with vitality that friends, family and yes, even doctors can see.

And trust me...

With this sugar secret and a healthy, low-carb diet in your arsenal—the health nags are going to stop giving you guff.

<u>That's a promise</u>.

With that boost in "watchdog enzyme" activity, you'll be armed with what I believe is...

"The first REAL breakthrough in sugar science in the past 100 years"

I don't think anyone has ever (and I mean EVER) experienced anything like it.

You're turning your body into a machine that faces the damaging effects of sugar head-on.

You're supercharging your system with a down-right force of nature that was made to keep you healthy. In the short amount of time that this natural discovery has been getting attention.

It's racked up quite a résumé...

It may put the brakes on damage brought on by excess glucose.

It may support and protect your blood vessels and could contribute to healthy blood vessel formation and repair.

Emerging research in animals shows it may help support the health of...

Kidney cells. Retina cells.

And beat the heck out of free radicals.

Imagine that—a brand new idea for defending against the damaging effects of sugar spikes.

It's a downright GIFT FROM GOD and—<u>it's a gift for YOU</u>.

You've waited long enough.

I've been a doctor for over 40 years and I must say, this is a bright-shining highlight in my medical career.

I've done my research and stayed ahead of the curve. So I'm proud to announce that not only have I heard of benfotiamine before most doctors—I've secured access to one HECK of a premium source.

And now I'm ready to let loose what is sure to be the most important formula I've ever created.

It's my personal BLOOD SUGAR BOMBSHELL.

I call it... **<u>GlucoComplete</u>**.

Honestly, I *wanted* to call it "Nag-Stop," but thought better of it at the last second...

Imagine, a cutting-edge breakthrough for blood sugar health.

You know what else is great? The smartest vitamin in existence—found in GlucoComplete... is an underground sensation.

And it's POWERFUL.

It's been used in Germany for a few years to support healthy nerve function, and it promotes the "watchdog enzyme" in your body that's 100 percent natural.

That's probably a big reason why benfotiamine has remained an "underground hero."

But with the 400 mg of benfotiamine found in every dose of GlucoComplete, you're taking steps to maintain healthy cells—kidney cells, retinal cells, and vascular cells—if glucose attacks.

So you can live with confidence. Live with comfort. And live with a little peace and quiet from all of the nagging...

And you know what?

GlucoComplete could stop with benfotiamine and I think it would still be all you need for the ultimate sugar support.

I'm serious, the way this discovery could help...

Your cells manage the effects of glucose that comes their way...

Protect your body from the dirty tricks of glucose...

And even promote your body's "watchdog enzyme"...

Honestly, I could have stopped with benfotiamine and you'd still have a revolutionary breakthrough on your hands—*but come on...*

Did Hank Aaron stop slamming home runs the day he broke the Babe's record? No...he piled on 50 more.

Did Edmund Hillary get halfway up Mount Everest and say, *"Eh, this is good enough."*

No!

You deserve a TRUE glucose game-changer

So while GlucoComplete could stop... <u>it goes even higher</u>.

And you know what's funny? The next blood sugar miracle found in GlucoComplete—couldn't be more different.

Where *benfotiamine* is an unbelievable underground sensation—this next secret in GlucoComplete has been boosting human health...for over 6,000 years.

Talk about "sufficient testing time..." But it gets even better—

If you can believe it, this natural hero is so reliable...so powerful...so overwhelming in popularity...even the USDA is researching it.

An *in vitro* study published in 2000 by the USDA itself showed that out of 49 botanical sugar secrets—this one demonstrated the greatest ability to support cellular glucose metabolism.

Heck, a current USDA research scientist is one of its biggest proponents.

Now all of that is well and good but this is a revolutionary formula we're talking about here.

You want to stop the nagging and maintain top-notch blood sugar control, right?

Of course you do.

That's why I've found an extract that's taken everything that's so special about this 6,000-year-old sugar secret...

And elevated it to brand new heights.

It's the aromatic spice, *cinnamon*. Now perhaps you've heard of cinnamon's blood sugar power before...

But trust me... you've never seen it like this before.

Cinnamon does a lot more than just make apple pie taste better.

It may also help your body support healthy blood sugar levels. And it's been shown *in vitro* to support glucose metabolism. Does that mean you should raid the spice rack to stop all the nagging?

You could... but I have something that's so much more powerful.

The secret that gives cinnamon such a powerful effect over insulin is a special compound called type-A polymers. And get a load of this...

Once they were discovered and isolated, these little buggers put up some heavy-duty results in vitro...

- **Type-A polymers have been shown to increase *in vitro* insulin activity 20 fold!**

- **They promote a healthy inflammatory response, they POUND free radical production and may help support cell membranes.**

Not only that...

- **They helped facilitate glucose metabolism and even aided glucose storage in fat cells.**

And the studies back it up...

In 2009, 22 healthy subjects took either 500 mg of these heavy-duty Type-A polymers or a placebo for 12 weeks, all while maintaining their normal eating and exercise habits.

While there weren't any significant changes in the placebo group at the end of the study, the cinnamon group was a different story...

Healthy blood glucose levels improved, as did oxidative stress levels..

And that was just with plain old cinnamon...

Imagine what you can do with this super-charged extract.

Let me show you...

A 12-week study conducted by the creators of this extract and using 22 subjects showed 500 mg of these polymers could help...

- Support healthy blood sugar levels...

- Maintain healthy systolic blood pressure levels...

And even...

- Decrease body fat

So you can see why these special polymers make cinnamon one super spice.

Now I could dash some cinnamon on top of the "sugar spike breakthrough" and call it a day. With that, you'd have the mightiest blood sugar support I've ever seen.

But this is GlucoComplete I'm talking about... there are plenty of formulas that might be happy doing that but...

Regular cinnamon isn't good enough for me and it certainly isn't good enough for you.

I know *type-A polymers* are the secret behind cinnamon's metabolic powers. So I hunted down...

The supernova of cinnamon extracts.

I've found a patented extract that's standardized for type-A polymers.

That means with every dose—you're guaranteed a potent punch of the very substance that makes cinnamon so special.

What if you could support healthy levels of blood sugar with ease?

What if you could maintain supreme blood sugar control throughout the years?

And what if you could finally...

Knock the naggers off their soapboxes?

GlucoComplete is rocketing 2 blood sugar juggernauts right into your bloodstream. You're helping to support your body's normal, healthy blood sugar levels and...

You're bolstering your body's levels of the "*glucose-guiding enzyme*"

It sounds too good to be true, right?

Just think...

Something NEW for your sugar support.

And not just *one* new breakthrough... but 2 bold, new approaches that would shock any doctor with their amazing blood sugar health abilities.

This is how you stop a nagger...

You prove that they don't know everything after all.

When they see what's inside your new sugar

support secret—I guarantee they'll scoff something like...

"*Well I've never heard of this before.*" Darn right, they haven't.

GlucoComplete is packed with only the best breakthroughs that will make naggers second-guess just how much they know to begin with.

That's good. That's step one.

Next... you back it up with proof.

Every day you're supplying your body with the power it needs to support premium blood sugar levels.

The nagging won't stop in one day... but little by little, they'll see your vitality... your ability to keep your blood sugar healthy and they'll think... "*Hmm... maybe he knows what he's talking about after all.*"

Can you imagine that? A little respect? A little confidence in the fact that you know what you're doing? And then suddenly...

The nagging just stops.

Imagine...

You can walk through your house without feeling like a lab rat—being prodded and inspected under a microscope.

It'll show. You can eat in peace, knowing that along with your healthy diet and some exercise, you've got that extra support helping to keep your blood sugar healthy naturally. You can go out with friends to your favorite restaurant and actually enjoy yourself, knowing that you're taking an additional step to complement your healthy diet and exercise routine.

And who knows—maybe you and that health nag in your life might actually start getting along a little better.

What I'm saying is...

You're not just helping keep your blood sugar levels in check... you're taking complete control over your health.

And I'm adding *one more* metabolic breakthrough into the mix.

Honestly, this final ingredient in GlucoComplete's revolutionary formula seals the deal on its potent power.

In fact, if you're currently taking anything at all to support normal, healthy blood sugar levels and it doesn't have this tried-and-true breakthrough—

I'm sorry... but you got a bust.

This miracle mineral is so well rounded...so complete... so tailor-made for sugar support...

I think of it as a—Blood Sugar Bulldozer. This one mineral may...

- **Help support healthy blood sugar levels...**

- **Be essential to the formation of glucose**

tolerance factor and...

• **Help support optimal insulin sensitivity so you get *the most* out of your body's natural glucose transporter.**

It was first discovered in the 50's and since then has shown positive results in more than a dozen human studies...

I'm talking about the mineral *chromium*. This mineral is perfect for promoting tighter blood sugar health and even with... the "sugar spike breakthrough" and the super charged 6,000-year-old sugar secret in its formula...

Well frankly, I wouldn't be able to call this breakthrough formula, GlucoComplete without it.

So I've infused chromium into every dose to create what could be...

The ULTIMATE breakthrough in natural blood sugar support

It's true—doctors, scientists and health nags around the world want to cram the same, *tired* ideas for blood sugar down your throat.

Imagine...

All of the stalling, all of the waiting, all of the *yap, yap, yap*...

COMES TO AN END TODAY.

So how does GlucoComplete work?

You're gonna like this...

All the cutting-edge blood sugar science found in GlucoComplete—

400 mg of the revolutionary benfotiamine...

500 mg of the supercharged cinnamon secret...

And the 200 mcg of the miracle mineral, chromium...

All fit into 2 of the tiniest capsules you'll ever see. There are no stinky horse pills here...

No gritty drinks, no fancy foods, no over-the-top solutions. That's one of the best parts—just how *easy* it is to give your blood sugar some extra support.

Now, you've seen solutions with a laundry list of ingredients... with puny amounts.

Is that how GlucoComplete works? Not on my watch.

Those other formulas are pushing a label—not providing you with support that works.

They load up a label with as many ingredients as they can to impress you and jack up the price—but you know better than to fall for those tricks. GlucoComplete provides you with 3 game-changing breakthroughs.

Nothing more, nothing less.

You get BIG AMOUNTS FOR BIG RESULTS.

I've done the research. I've tirelessly looked for decades.

These 3 breakthroughs are what you need for confident blood sugar support. And I'm not going to bog it down with unnecessary ingredients to drive up the price tag.

And GlucoComplete is designed to give you new discoveries that you've never seen before. The kind that'll have the health nags scratching their scalps and questioning how much they really knew to begin with.

And do these natural breakthroughs come with a hefty price tag? That might be the greatest news of all—but first, I want to make one more promise to you.

When you start taking this revolutionary approach to blood sugar support...

When you start powering your body with nutrients it needs to protect you from the ravaging effects of glucose spikes...

When you help support your own natural insulin sensitivity and maintain a healthy, low-carb diet...

You're going to see results FAST.

Remember: You should visit your doctor regularly to have your blood sugar tested. Inform him that you are taking a supplement that could have an effect on your blood sugar levels. If he is our kind of doctor, he will appreciate it.

In fact... let me spell it out. Take the health nag in your life...

It could be your wife. Your kids. Even your doctor.

And then give it 6 weeks.

That's right...

Just 6 weeks and notice how quiet your house becomes. You can walk through the kitchen without being bombarded with questions. You can watch the nightly news without getting a lecture at every commercial break.

And how about this...

NOT HEAR ONE WORD ABOUT IT.

So what do you think?

Are you ready to grab the reins of your health?

Are you ready to silence the nagging once and for all?

Are you ready to experience something exciting for blood sugar support? Visit the Wellness Directory on page 409 for ordering information.

Chapter 36:

Cut Your Diabetes Risk by 83 Percent by Choosing the Right Beverages

And now for more inane and superfluous news, hot off the press of the American Medical Association: Women who drink higher amounts of sugar-sweetened drinks are more likely to gain weight and develop Type II diabetes, "new" research tells us. New? Seems to me I learned that 40 years ago.

The study supposedly adds "new fuel to the debate" on the sources of weight gain and their ultimate impact on the ever-growing diabetes epidemic. I don't see any "new fuel" here but some of the "old fuel" bears further inspection since Type II diabetes and its "partner," obesity are having a bull run.

Reuters Health reports: "According to the study authors, soft drinks are the leading source of added sugars in the U.S. diet. Moreover, the increase in the prevalence of diabetes and obesity has coincided with a 61 percent increase in the consumption of soft drinks by adults, and a doubling in consumption by children and adolescents between the late 1970s and the mid-1990s."

Don't fall for diet

Of course, true to AMA form, they went off on a tangent that had nothing to do with the rest of the study (but undoubtedly distracted enough "experts" to take the heat off sugar for a minute). In this study, women who drank high levels of sugar-sweetened soft drinks "also smoked more, were less physically active, and had lower intakes of fiber and magnesium." Ah ha, now we're getting to the bottom of things: How do you measure all that? You do it by interviewing the patient, which is known to be notoriously inaccurate and worthless. And before I forget to ask, what does smoking have to do with diabetes and obesity? The experts are saying that obesity causes diabetes. Well since smoking prevents weight gain, then how can it cause diabetes? But back to the real issue.

"Even after adjusting for other factors, women who consumed one or more sugar-sweetened soft drinks per day had an 83 percent increased risk of developing diabetes compared to those who drank less than one per month. Diet cola and fruit juice were not associated with Type II diabetes." This report on diet cola is misleading and dangerous. The artificial sweetener in "diet" drinks has been accused of its own misdeeds including weight gain and Parkinson's disease.

The right treatment makes all the difference.

There is a commonly held belief among nutritionists and medical scientists that fatness is a causative factor in the onset of diabetes. I'm not so sure, but Doctor JoAnn Manson, a study co-author and a professor of medicine at Harvard Medical School, remarked: "High-fructose corn syrup leads to fast and dramatic rises in glucose and insulin levels, and that can lead to insulin resistance and the development of Type II diabetes."

"About half of the increase in the risk of Type II diabetes is due to the weight gain that occurs with sugar-sweetened beverages, but the other half may be related to the fact that these sugars are rapidly absorbable," said Dr. Manson.

As I mentioned above, I don't necessarily agree that fatness by itself leads to diabetes. But there is an important message here that I will put in terms everyone can understand.

The rapid increase in blood sugar as a result of drinking a massive dose of corn syrup (the main sweetener in soda) leads to a rapid increase of the insulin secreted by the pancreas into the blood. Ordinarily, insulin will metabolize the extra sugar, bringing the blood sugar level back to normal. But if you keep drinking the stuff and placing constant demands on the insulin-secreting cells in the pancreas, eventually the insulin just doesn't work anymore.

Action to take:

Some doctors (those so-called experts again) "treat" this problem by having the patient give himself insulin shots. But adding more insulin to insulin-saturated blood will not solve the problem. The only solution is to eliminate sugar and sugar-forming foods—starches. That's right, not just cut back on them, but stop eating them altogether. Sugary drinks are a good place to start, but that's all it is—a start.

Chapter 37:

Your Guide to Beating One of Today's Leading Killers... CURE DIABETES IN THREE EASY STEPS

Lies, lies and more lies—if you're diabetic, you hear the lies every single day, starting with the biggest whopper of them all: You can't cure diabetes.

All you can do is take your meds, pump yourself full of insulin, switch to a miserable high-carb low-fat diet, cross your fingers, and hope for the best, according to standard mainstream "medical" advice.

Just ask anyone on that plan how well it's working out.

If you're on it yourself, you already know the answer—and if you keep at it, you'll get fatter and sicker until you medicate yourself right into an early grave.

Well, it's time for some truth instead of lies—because despite what you've heard, you don't need to live with this disease.

And you're certainly not doomed to die of it.

There's another way—a BETTER way—and now, even the U.S. government has (in its own way) admitted that I've been right all along on this: The best and only way to cure diabetes isn't with a drug at all.

It's with diet.

(Don't worry; I'd never suggest you start shoving what the mainstream calls "a diet" down your throat. More on that in a moment...)

In a new CDC study of close to 4,500 diabetics, the agency found that intensive counseling—counseling sessions so constant they bordered on nagging—helped 11.5 percent reverse diabetes to the point where they were no longer diabetic.

They were now considered "pre" diabetic, and some of them were actually cured.

That's right—**CURED**, and not a drug in sight.

Now, 11.5 percent might sound like a low success rate, but it's not because weight loss doesn't work for everyone. It's because many people simply won't commit to weight loss no matter how much you nag them.

And that's why your own plan to beat diabetes MUST begin in one place...

STEP ONE:
LOSE THE WEIGHT

Weight loss should be the number one goal of any diabetic—and in the new CDC study, the people who lost the most weight were 20 percent more likely to go into remission than those who didn't lose much.

Clearly, you want to shed some pounds—lots of pounds, because the more you lose, the better your chances.

The real problem with the new study is that the CDC (and every other mainstream medical group) backs the wrong horse when it comes to diet. They're still harping on low-fat, and that's exactly how you DON'T lose weight.

The proof is in the fat-free pudding: Dieters in the new CDC study who went to the nag sessions lost 8.6 percent of their body weight. Nothing to sneeze at, but not the life-changing weight loss you need to get the job done, either.

If you want REAL results and a REAL shot at success, try a REAL diet instead—one that's scientifically proven to lead to both weight loss and improvements in every major diabetes risk factor.

<u>STEP TWO:</u>
SWITCH TO A HIGH-FAT, LOW-CARB DIET

Now you've heard me sing the praises of this lifestyle plenty of times before. But if you're diabetic, it's not optional.

For you, a low-carb, high-fat diet ***is a matter of survival***.

Carb control is essential to blood sugar control—and along with weight loss, blood sugar control is critical to beating this disease.

In one recent study, a diet of even 20 percent carbs reduced the need for insulin in diabetics by nearly a third. In another, a diet of just 10 percent carbs not only improved insulin sensitivity, but it also kicked the body into a higher gear for weight loss.

People who were able to keep their carb consumption below that threshold **burned 350 calories MORE each day** than low-fat dieters eating the same number of calories.

That's equivalent to a painful hour of exercise in the gym every day—without spilling a drop of sweat, risking injury, or paying sky-high gym membership fees.

With a body operating that efficiently, of course you'll lose plenty of weight—but don't stop with weight loss, because there's one other step you need to take... one that can mean the difference between success and failure.

And no one else is talking about this one yet.

STEP THREE:
BALANCE YOUR BELLY

There are more than three pounds of bacteria sitting in your gut right now—a mix of the good bugs needed for digestion and health and the bad ones that are constantly trying to undermine them.

This balance—or, in too many cases, *lack* of

balance—is what will either keep you healthy or bring on disease. And diabetes is one of the key diseases linked to gut imbalances in emerging research.

In one recent study out of China, diabetics were consistently found to have an overload of bad gut bacteria when compared to non-diabetics. In other studies, we've seen why: Good bacteria produce the hormones and other biochemicals needed to ward off diabetes in the first place.

If you don't have these good bugs, you could do everything right and still end up in a fight for your life with a chronic disease.

And odds are, your own supply of good bugs is dwindling right now whether you have diabetes or not.

Poor diet and antibiotics—the ones you've taken intentionally as well as the ones hidden in your food and drink—are a one-two punch in the belly that wipe out the good bugs you need and give the bad ones a chance to take control.

Minimize your antibiotic exposure by switching to organic meats, and filter your water with reverse osmosis (and only take the darned drugs when you actually need them).

Then, give the good guys in your gut some reinforcements by taking a quality probiotic supplement each day.

Follow these three steps, and success is practically guaranteed. I know that sounds simple—but let's be honest here. If it really was that simple, you wouldn't be obese and diabetic in the first place.

But forget how you got here. It's time to look ahead, not back—time to get started on a path to a drug-free life where diabetes is something you used to have.

You can do it—but you had better get started right now. The longer you wait, the harder it'll be.

And eventually, we all run out of time.

Chapter 38:

The Nutrition Lesson 100 Years in the Making: Learn It Now and Stay Diabetes-Free for Good

Well it's about time. It is hard to believe that it took 100 years for the diet dictators, those of food pyramid fame, to face the obvious, which is: Diabetes is caused by an excessive intake of sugar—period.

According to the report I read, "corn syrup and other refined foods may be much to blame for the huge increase in type-2 diabetes in the United States over the past few decades..." You look at the simple nutritional facts and it seems unbelievable that the university experts could be so blind for so long. But it's not so surprising if you understand the simple economics of the thing: The people who pay the bills at the various university research institutions set up the base of the food pyramid. But the grains and starches that make up the base turn to sugar in your blood, and that turns into gold for the junk food industry.

But maybe the "experts" are finally starting to catch on: "A study of nearly 100 years of data on what Americans eat show a huge increase in processed carbohydrates, especially corn syrup..." reports *Reuters*.

Lee Gross, author of the study, said he was not "picking on the corn syrup industry," but added, "it is hard to ignore the fact that 20 percent of our carbohydrates are coming from corn syrup—10 percent of our total calories."

Gross, with colleagues at the Harvard School of Public Health and the CDC, found that starting in 1980 people began consuming steadily more calories, with an average increase in total calories of 500 a day. It's hardly a coincidence that the number of packaged, corn-syrup-laden foods on the supermarket shelves has also gone up in the same time frame.

Gross' solution to this ballooning problem pays homage to fruits and vegetables, while <u>completely ignoring</u> the major components in food that make you healthy and diabetes-free: animal fat and animal protein. By ignoring these keys to good health, he's just contributing to the great food pyramid hoax that has led to the diabetic epidemic we are in.

Corny excuses

Audrae Erickson, president of the Corn Refiners Association, called the report "misleading." (They always say that when some researcher has the audacity to point the finger at sugar.)

"Diabetes rates are rising in many countries

around the world that use little or no high fructose corn syrup in foods and beverages... the primary causes of diabetes are obesity, advancing age and heredity," she said. This statement is just a sampling of the misleading and irrelevant claptrap we get from the sugar industry.

Obesity does not cause diabetes, and diabetes does not cause obesity. They are <u>both</u> caused by the excessive intake of SUGAR and starch-related substandard foods.

"Advancing age" is not a disease but a reward for leading a life with good nutrition. And it does not lead to diabetes unless you brought it on yourself through a high-sugar diet.

Heredity is not the issue here either. That is only a problem in childhood (type 1) diabetes, where the child is <u>genetically deficient</u> in factors that control blood sugar. Less than 5 percent of diabetics come under this hereditary classification. "Heredity" is a red herring in this argument, and Erickson knows that.

So you see how the sugar lobby tries to manipulate you? Sure, Al Quaeda is an enemy worth close attention, but don't let it distract you from the government, the university nutrition obfuscators, Big Sugar, and the press—they're <u>all</u> your enemies.

Chapter 39:

Could You Be the Next Victim of Syndrome X, or—Even Worse—Syndrome H?

...for hype. I apologize (again) for being such a cynic, but is this <u>really</u> a new syndrome or just a clever propaganda ploy to cover up the fact that Americans have been misled as to why they are overweight and sick from diabetes? Oh sure, not all diabetics are fat. But <u>all</u> diabetics are seriously ill from a form of iatrogenesis I call "Syndrome Z" (just to twit the so-called experts). Iatrogenesis is any disease that is caused by physicians—in this case ones who have been giving bad—and in many cases, fatal—nutrition advice for two generations.

The gist of the latest report says that a new disease, called "insulin resistance syndrome" has been discovered. But that's too boring to really capture the public's attention, so they're also calling it "Syndrome X" and warning us that it "can develop into diabetes as well as heart disease, nonalcoholic fatty liver and perhaps some cancers such as colon and ovarian cancer."

The adult disease our children
are catching

At a recent news conference, Dr. Daniel Einhorn of the Scripps Whittier Institute for Diabetes in La Jolla, California, said "As the prevalence of insulin resistance syndrome has skyrocketed 61 percent in the last decade, it is crucial that medical professionals have consistent and definitive criteria to assess this serious condition."

To be "consistent" and "definitive," why not call it what it is: <u>adult onset diabetes</u> (type II diabetes)? But the sad fact is that it's not just adults anymore—it's now being seen in young adults and children. Apparently, pediatricians are starting to see obesity and type 2 diabetes in an increasing number of 7- to 10-year olds.

<u>Exactly</u>!

The pediatricians have (for once) hit the nail on the head: It's not Syndrome This or Syndrome That—it's adult onset diabetes in <u>children</u>. It's that simple.

Treating diabetes:
A little doesn't always go a long way

So what can people do to treat their new "syndrome"? Here Dr. Einhorn adds to the confusion by saying that a little weight loss and a little exercise "will help a good deal," which is highly doubtful. And then he goes the last mile for the junk food cartel: "It is not necessary to cut out all sweets," he added. According to the article I read, "like many doctors, Einhorn does not believe claims that carbohydrates are to blame for obesity."

Well, I have news for you, Daniel, <u>it is absolutely vital</u> that people with this condition, whether you call it "Syndrome X" or by its real name—DIABETES—<u>avoid all sugar and starch (carbohydrates) in their diet</u>. Any advice less stringent than this is a disservice to the patient, bordering on malpractice.

And he says <u>carbohydrates aren't to blame</u> for obesity? Einhorn must not read *The New York Times*. Someone should tell him that the fat vs. carbs war is over and that even *The Times*, the purveyor of bad advice, both political and nutritional, for 75 years, has capitulated and admitted that fat doesn't make you fat. And it's not "genetics" or "modern living" per se, Dr. Einhorn. Sugar and starch—<u>carbohydrates</u>—have caused the fattening and "diabeticizing" of America—right down to our children.

Chapter 40:

Considering Knee Surgery? Read This First! 7 Keys to Beating Ostearthritis Without Drugs or Surgery

---

There are two kinds of people battling the pain of knee osteoarthritis: those who think they need surgery... and those who've already had it.

The dirty secret of the orthopedic industry is that those surgeries rarely end the pain or improve movement, and they can even leave you in more agony than ever.

If you don't believe me, ask anyone who went through the expensive surgery and struggled through the long and painful recovery only to discover that their "new" knees are no better than the old creaky ones.

And if you already learned the hard way yourself, you can rest assured that you're not alone. Your surgery didn't "fail." It went exactly as could have been predicted or even expected—because there's precious little evidence to back most knee procedures, and plenty of evidence against them.

Randomized studies in both 2002 and 2008 found absolutely no benefit for the wildly popular arthroscopic surgery for knee osteoarthritis patients, including **_no difference in pain, physical function, and quality of life_**. None!

Some doctors are now doing fewer of these procedures, but it's not because they've realized the error of their ways. It's because they've found something even more profitable—and even less proven. They call it the total knee replacement, but I call it...

The joint scam of the 21st century.

Total knee replacements are spreading like wildfire, with some 600,000 of them performed each year in the United States alone. But earlier this year, a study in *Lancet* found little evidence to back the safety, effectiveness, and even patient satisfaction with the procedure.

Even worse, many of the 30 or 40 replacement knees on the market have been poorly tested or not tested at all, thanks to lax regulations for implanted devices (including a tasty loophole that allows new medical devices to be approved with practically no testing if the maker claims it's basically the same as an existing approved model... even if it's not).

No wonder they're being recalled almost as frequently as automobiles—and you can bet your "good" knee this is only the beginning, because there are more consumer protections in place over car parts than there are for body parts.

But in spite of all that, your orthopedist is still making promises he can't keep and giving you the hard sell for surgery.

If you want to know why, don't look at the evidence... as I just explained, it's not there. Look at his home. Find it on Google Earth if you can. Pay close attention to the size of his palace... the big swimming pool... and his fleet of luxury cars. You'd think he was a Wall Street fat cat.

Orthopedic surgeons are the highest paid doctors in the nation. They make double the salary of the average family doctor, and many make several times that. And let's face it, they don't get those big piles of cash by NOT operating.

Well, dear reader, the jig is up—because I'm here to tell you that while you might not be able to cure osteoarthritis pain in the knees and elsewhere, you sure can do a heck of a lot better than you're doing now.

And you don't need drugs OR surgery—just my seven steps to success:

1) Cod Liver Oil: Think of it as lubricant for your joints. It's a time-tested remedy long known for its anti-inflammatory properties, and (unlike replace-ment knees) it's backed by research: A 2002 study from Cardiff University found that cod liver oil slashed levels of the enzyme responsible for joint cartilage damage in osteoarthritis patients, and that the effect was noticeable in as little as 24

hours. The longer you take it, the greater the benefit—so start today.

2) Glucosamine and Chondroitin: Your orthopedist will tell you these two don't work. He's lying because, unlike the surgery he's pushing, glucosamine and chondroitin are backed by both science and the testimonials of the millions of people who rely on them for osteoarthritis relief. A series of studies out of Belgium showed that this dynamic duo can bring pain relief and reverse the joint calcification that marks the condition. They can also ease stiffness and restore motion. The downside is that it can take a few weeks or even a few months to kick in—but I promise you, it's worth the wait.

3) Curcumin: It's the spice that gives curry its color—and a 2010 study found it's as effective as ibuprofen at pain relief for osteoarthritis. Ibuprofen, of course, can wreck your stomach or even punch a hole right through it. Curry is delicious. You tell me which is the better option.

4) Devil's Claw: Sounds like something I made up to see if you're still paying attention, but devil's claw isn't something mixed with eye of newt and bat's breath. It's a traditional herbal remedy—and a 2002 study found it could match the pain relief and mobility benefits of the European drug diacerein, with none of the risks. Now that's giving the devil his due!

5) Lose Weight: All our knees wear down as we age. But if you're asking your hinges to support a super-sized frame, they're not just going to wear down—they're going to break down. A study last year found that losing weight improved pain, stiffness, physical function, and overall quality of life in knee osteoarthritis patients. All I can say is, no kidding.

6) Quit Exercise: If you're going to the gym, demand a refund—and if you've been jogging or running, quit before it's too late. The best way to wreck your joints—especially your knees—is by constantly taxing them through exercise such as running and lifting. You should still make sure you get out and stay mobile, just do it with safer activities such as walking, bicycling, golf, or even gardening instead.

7) Smoke Like a Chimney: You read that right! It might not be politically correct, but the nicotine in tobacco protects joints from osteoarthritis damage and may even prevent the disease from occurring in the first place. One recent study of 11,388 senior Australian men found that longtime smokers were up to 51 percent less likely to need a total joint replacement than nonsmokers. I recommend a quality cigar after meals. No, you don't have to inhale; cigar smokers don't inhale. The nutrients from cigar smoke are absorbed by the mucous membranes of the mouth.

So while all your friends end up stoned on narcotic drugs for pain relief after failed knee surgeries, you'll be out teeing off on the golf course with a stogie—enjoying life. And isn't that how your golden years are supposed to be?

Chapter 41:

Return to the Days of Healthy Joints and Muscles

As you get older, it gets harder and harder to live a normal life without having many of the things you've done for years be disrupted by pain. Your joints, back, hands, elbows, shoulders, knees, hips—you name it—all start to ache.

Go to your doctor and chances are he'll give you nonsteroidal anti-inflammatory drugs (NSAIDs)—drugs like ibuprofen (Advil) and naprosyn (Aleve)—to treat chronic joint and skeletal pain.

NSAIDs work by attacking a class of natural biochemical called prostaglandins. These essential body chemicals cause inflammation but also aid in healing.

By attacking them, NSAIDs destroy the body's natural healing agents. So when you take NSAIDs, you may temporarily mask the pain, but you do nothing to treat the underlying condition.

What doctors either gloss over or don't tell

you at all is that NSAIDs are far from safe.
Their side effects are well documented in pub-
lications like *The American Journal of Medicine* (May 31, 1999) and *The Physicians' Desk
Reference*, the "bible" of prescription drugs.

The side effects of NSAIDs can include nausea, an upset stomach, bleeding ulcers, constipation, diarrhea, depression, headache, dizziness, mental confusion, and hair loss.

Fortunately, there are a handful of alternative therapies that are proven to be safe and
effective.

A 60-year-old secret relieves pain by treating the source, not the symptoms

Unlike drugs, prolotherapy gets to the source
of your joint, tendon, and muscle pain. And it
doesn't cause side effects.

In a nutshell, prolotherapy calls on your
body's resources to rebuild damaged parts.

First, the prolotherapist injects a safe solution, usually containing dextrose (a simple
sugar) and lidocaine (a topical anesthetic),
right into the damaged, painful area. The solution causes a slight amount of inflammation
at the injection site. This may not sound too
good, but, in fact, the inflammation is the basis of the treatment and is the first phase of a
three-stage process of healing.

Inflammation is a sign of two natural body-repair mechanisms, white blood cells and prostaglandins, working at the site of the damage. Increased blood flow to the area brings white blood cells to remove damaged tissue.

The injected solution also attracts prostaglandins, one of your body's natural healers, and sets the stage for the second phase of healing.

Be advised that this first stage is accompanied by increased swelling and sometimes increased pain, which lasts about a week. It is the most difficult stage for first-time users of prolotherapy. Instead of experiencing the immediate (but short-lived) relief that painkillers give, the condition may seem to get a little worse. If necessary, prolotherapists usually recommend taking acetaminophen and applying some ice to the painful area. (Or try a few cubes in a glass of whiskey.)

After about a week, the second phase—known as the fibroblastic stage—begins. During this stage, specialized cells called fibroblasts build connective tissue, thus repairing the damage from your injury. Pain and swelling subside, and new blood vessels are built. This stage lasts between two and four weeks.

The third and final phase of healing, the maturation stage, occurs at around week six and continues for up to two years after the onset of treatment. During this stage, the new blood vessels mature and new tissue becomes stronger.

Dr. George Hackett, considered the "father of prolotherapy," spent many years researching this treatment and published his results in a groundbreaking monograph and in *The Journal of the American Medical Association*.

Hackett's results showed that after prolotherapy, underlying connective tissue increases in size and strength by as much as 40 percent.

Some pain can be taken care of in one prolotherapy treatment. However, most cases of chronic pain will take two to 10 sessions for optimal pain relief to occur. When more than one session is necessary, injections are given at one-week intervals, although the interval between injections depends on the area and the severity of pain and can be as long as six weeks.

According to the research of Dr. Tom Dorman of the Paracelsus Clinic in Washington, approximately 90 percent of the people treated with prolotherapy will experience between 50 percent and 100 percent pain relief.

With results this promising, you may be wondering why you haven't heard of prolotherapy. Mainly, because it's not taught in medical schools. It is also not covered by most insurance companies. The insurance companies and the American Medical Association classify prolotherapy as "investigative" and "experimental." And, finally, drug companies make a lot of money on prescriptions and surgeons make just as much performing surgeries for conditions that could be effectively and cheaply treated by prolotherapy. They don't want this treatment to gain mainstream status. There is just too much at stake for them.

Action to take:

You can contact the American Association of Orthopedic Medicine at (800) 992-2063, or online at www.aaomed.org for a list of doctors who practice prolotherapy.

Harness your body's healing power for strong and supple joints

You won't hear this from your average HMO-sponsored orthopedist (who's probably so young he doesn't have to worry about his joints himself), but the key to life-long joint health—even long into your twilight years—isn't masking joint discomfort with drugs or temporarily "zapping" them with steroids. No, you need to keep them nourished from the start.

By nourishing them from the inside out with the proper nutrients and antioxidants, your joints can actually maintain themselves, giving you the kind of strength, mobility and range of motion you've always enjoyed. But believe me, it's not as simple as stopping by the grocery store and stocking up on discount vitamins.

The best way to "turn back the clock" for your joints is a powerful nutrient attack that:

• Keeps joints moving

• Naturally helps build cartilage for greater flexibility and mobility

• Infuses your joints with powerful antioxidants

By far one of the most important nutrients for joints is a molecule called **methylsulfonyl-methane (MSM)**.

MSM is what supplies our bodies with sulfur, a vital element for healthy joints that's absolutely crucial to the regeneration of cells—especially cartilage.

MSM by helping your body regenerate healthy new cells to replace the old, worn and torn ones in your cartilage.

And, of course, you can't talk about joint health without discussing glucosamine. Glucosamine is a name you hear all the time when it comes to keeping joints healthy. But is just any old glucosamine sufficient to make your joints healthy and strong once again? And, does it *have* to be paired with chondroitin? The answer is "no"—on both accounts.

For it to be effective at increasing your strength and flexibility, it has to be the *right* kind of glucosamine. Glucosamine sulfate is the closest thing available to the glucosamine your body makes on its own for good joint health.

The benefits of glucosamine have been shown time and again—in studies, clinical trials, and in years of use by millions of consumers.

Yes, glucosamine sulfate is phenomenally effective for joint health. It can promote generation of healthy, new cartilage and address concerns of stiffness and discomfort.

Though it may take a few weeks to kick in, its effects are real, long lasting, and accumulate over time.

But, what about chondroitin?

Chondroitin is often combined with glucosamine in joint formulations because they have been shown to work well together in protecting joints. However, some studies have shown that chondroitin may play a part in the spread of prostate cancer. While the jury is still out on this, I would recommend staying away from chondroitin. Plenty of studies show that glucosamine is effective on its own—so what's the point of putting yourself at risk?

Action to take:

MSM and glucosamine are readily available at most health food stores, some pharmacies, and even grocery stores. I recommend 750 mg of MSM and 1,500 mg of glucosamine.

The joint health discovery no one saw coming

It could come as a quick creak in your wrist or give you some trouble after an afternoon hike. Or it could happen on the back nine as you raise your club and your elbow starts to twitch. Or even crouching in your garden when you feel like your knees and hips don't want to let you back up...

Any one of these moments, the culprit might not be what you think. It's not your fault— we've been programmed to assume the trouble *must be* in our joints.

So for ages (forever, really)—that's all anyone has bothered to focus on. But what do those head-scratchers think is holding all of your joints together???

I know my medical school taught me this... **TENDONS.**

And for the first time *ever*, there's finally a *real* solution that addresses tendon health

Because until now, even if you were lucky enough to know it was your tendons... (and believe me, a lot of people *don't* know.) Once your tendons underwent everyday wear and tear, there wasn't much anyone could tell you to do besides apply some ice, rest and maybe do some stretches.

Stretches??? **I've seen better advice come out of a fortune cookie!**

They might as well hand you a lollipop, too. IT'S JUST NOT GOOD ENOUGH... not by a long shot. But that ends today.

Today, there's finally a breakthrough way that has the potential to keep your tendons healthy and on the move. A way to protect and support your tendons so you can help keep them active. I found something my colleagues weren't even looking for. It's an advanced way to support your tendon health so you can keep going without worrying about every twinge, tweak and ache...

You see, the only time you're likely to hear

anything about tendons is when you turn on ESPN and see the latest player carted to the sidelines. Heck, they even give tendon injuries sports names like "Tennis" or "Golfer's Elbow." But you don't have to be some muscled-up hulk for your tendons to strike you down.

And it doesn't take an injury for your tendons to act up either. Normal everyday reaching, bending, picking-up and grabbing can be all it takes. Because the repetitive motions you make in your day-to-day life can be especially stressful for tendons...

Things like typing or scrubbing dishes—or even daily walks can put extra strain on your tendons. **Literally every single move you make uses your tendons.**

For instance, you've probably heard of the Achilles' tendon. But that's only 1 of over **4,000** tendons you've got throughout your entire body. And each of them needs to be in tip-top shape to help keep you moving free and easy. Which is why this discovery means so much.

For the first time, there's actually a way to support your tendons naturally. Now you can help take control of your tendon health, rather than sitting around waiting helplessly. You see, tendons have been misunderstood for a *very long* time. And I'm not surprised if you're looking for some answers...

Tendons are tough, flexible bands, made mostly of collagen, that connect your muscles to your bones. They're kind of like internal rubber bands that keep your muscles, bones and joints in place so you can move the way you were built to. And just like rubber bands, they can only be stretched so far and so many times before they start to give.

And boy, will you _feel_ it if they do...

And that's not all—as you age, even if you're not really that active, your tendons start to lose their elasticity, which could leave you feeling stiff. But the problem is, once your tendons are in trouble, they take a very long time to recover.

It could be months... Which is a shameful disgrace!

But unlike other doctors, I didn't just sit around waiting for someone else to figure it out. I decided to find a different approach...

You see, tendons are much more vital to your mobility and comfort than most people (*and obviously most doctors*) realize.

Try this: Hold out your hand straight in front of you and close your fingers and thumb into a fist—*You just used at least 38 tendons*.

And if just one of them is acting up—that simple motion is NOT so simple. And that's just the tendons in your hand. Tendons stretch up and down your arms and legs. Tendons keep your hips and shoulders in their sockets. They're in your neck and back, they're in your elbows, your knees, your feet, fingers, wrists and toes...

And over time, just through normal use—your tendons can take quite a beating.

Just think about every move you make throughout the day—walking, writing, sitting, standing, driving. All of these motions involve the thousands of tendons you've got supporting your joints, muscles and bones, so after years of bending and flexing your tendons countless times—it's easy to understand why you might start to feel their wear. But why put yourself through that?

Why assume it's your joints just because that's all the mainstream ever talks about?

No matter what they say, you don't have to give up the active lifestyle you've always enjoyed.

Because the hidden reason *nothing* seems to give your joints the support they need... whether it's the tweaks and aches you worry about when kneeling down at the ninth hole or gardening...

All of it could mean—**It's your tendons.**

That's why I want to tell you about a unique way to take action now. Today, I'm catapulting tendon health out of the Stone Age and into the 21st century.

Now there's finally something to keep your tendons healthy, strong and ready to go. Something to keep your tendons moving and comfortable— whether you're on the golf course, gardening or just cooking dinner.

And today, I'm proud to introduce it to you. It's the only natural solution in existence I know of that focuses directly on your tendons, your comfort and your mobility. And I bet it'll be the most triumphant tendon breakthrough in the whole history of medicine.

Because after months of digging through all the research I could get my hands on...

I finally found the answer
I was looking for in Europe

During my search, one of my sources gave me the word about a group of daring researchers trying a new approach to tendon health. So I looked into it right away—combing over and questioning all the details and reports, page after page.

And there it was, plain as day. Almost as if it was waiting for me to come along and tell the whole world about it. Those researchers weren't just onto something... they had the beginnings of an all-out scientific breakthrough on their hands...

So I contacted them right away and luckily, my reputation preceded me. And we started working together immediately to bring this revolutionary formula to the U.S.

And it's something I think holds the potential to shake the health community to its core. Because this could finally be the way to **safe-**

guard your tendons now and forever.

And once you know this unique way to support your tendon health, you can keep moving and save all that ice for your scotch. I've got to say, I chucked a lot of other ideas into the "NO" pile before I found this one...

This is just so unlike anything else because this solution sends aid straight to the source—**right to your tendons.**

So I called it **Ultimate Tendon Support.**

And the reason this formula is so different— is how it works. I mentioned earlier how your tendons are made of collagen and that over time, with constant use, they can start to weaken, **since every move you make puts stress on your tendons.**

But Ultimate Tendon Support goes toe-to-toe with that concern by giving you the nutrients your body needs to support healthy tendons. You see, tendons are notoriously hard to nourish because they're mostly avascular. That means they have a very limited blood supply and in some spots—they have no access to your bloodstream at all.

So unlike other areas of your body, you just can't rely on nutrients being delivered through your bloodstream. And while others threw in the towel, I found a different way to give your tendons the support they need.

You see, the trick *isn't* giving your tendons the special nutrients. That would be nice but your bloodstream just doesn't make enough "stops" at your tendons. So the way to do it is, give your body the nutrients it uses to build healthy tendons in the first place.

And thanks to the groundbreaking formula at the center of Ultimate Tendon Support, now you can. It's called TendoFit™—and it's a special dual-action blend of two essential tendon-supporting nutrients.

The first nutrient is so impressive, scientists came up with quite a name for it: Mucopolysaccharides (MPS).

Remember how I mentioned earlier that your tendons are made up of tough bands of collagen...

Well, MPS is kind of like the glue holding all those bands together. So you need proper levels of MPS in your tendons, so they stay strong.

Because MPS helps keep the structure of your tendons strong and intact and keeping you on the move. So you can see that making sure you've got plenty of MPS is a key part of supporting healthy tendons.

But that's not all it does. While MPS works hard to keep your tendons strong—it'll work overtime to support your joint cartilage. Because MPS also makes up about 20 percent of your cartilage and has even been found to help promote joint comfort and mobility.

In fact, most of the research on MPS to date has been completely focused on joint health. And now we know it's also one of the greatest nutrients you can give your tendons, too.

But TendoFit is just getting warmed up. It's a dual-acting formula. And it was the second ingredient that had me out of my chair, pacing circles around my desk as I read about it in excitement.

It's something we've all heard of but I was shocked to discover that it's never been used like this before

Type 1 Collagen.

I'm sure you've heard of it, but collagen has far better uses than plumping the lips of Hollywood starlets. **In fact, there are at least 28 distinct types of collagen in your body**. And while they all have similar functions—they're NOT all the same. Some are much stronger than others, for example.

You see, your tendons are made of about 70 percent collagen and 95 percent of that collagen is Type 1. And that's important, because when it comes to your tendons—the type of collagen inside them makes all the difference.

In fact, one study found that as we put more strain on our tendons, our bodies start producing more Type 3 and less Type 1. And this can cause all sorts of problems...

You see, Type 3 is much weaker than Type 1

and it is much harder for it to handle the kind of force and stress your tendons take on a daily basis. Because while the *structure* of your tendons relies on MPS, the strength of your tendons depends on their collagen content. And they depend specifically on Type 1. Which is why Type 1 collagen makes the perfect partner to MPS.

Plus, just like MPS, Type 1 collagen supports your cartilage, too. In addition to making up 70 percent of your tendons, Type 1 collagen is also responsible for maintaining the structure of your joint cartilage.

Meaning TendoFit's double dose of tendon nutrients may just be the next generation in cartilage care, too.

This research looked great on paper but I insist on seeing real-life results before I recommend anything. And I couldn't be happier to say, preliminary research on TendoFit shows very promising results.

Because this special blend of MPS and Type 1 collagen was put to the test in Europe. The researchers that developed TendoFit conducted an unpublished, in vitro trial. That just means it's one of those experiments with little petri dishes you see all the time on the science channel.

And they found that TendoFit could help **stimulate the production of <u>NEW</u> tendon cells.**

Now, since this trial was performed on cells it used a higher concentration of TendoFit than can be packed into a supplement. But those new tendon cells didn't just magically appear. It was the TendoFit that gave them the extra help they needed.

So it was clear to me from the start that these findings weren't just promising—they were groundbreaking!

Then, on the heels of this study, the manufacturer wanted to see how TendoFit worked for people complaining about their tendons. So they conducted another unpublished small study using people who felt discomfort in their tendons.

In this preliminary study, all 80 participants were required to attend physical therapy sessions two to three times a week but only half of them were also given TendoFit.

Then both groups were assessed in two ways. First, all participants took surveys after 3 months. And the TendoFit group described more improvement than the control group.

It was great to hear from people saying it worked but the researchers went a step further...

And asked a physiotherapist to examine everyone's tendon comfort, too. And again, the lucky group testing TendoFit **showed more improvement than the control group**...

After 30 days... the TendoFit group was doing noticeably better than the control group.

After 60 days... the TendoFit group was doing even better...

And finally... after 90 days... yep, you guessed it... the TendoFit group measured even better than the control group.

And that's after just 3 months! That's an unheard of supersonic pace when it comes to tendons...

But the best finding of all was listed last in the report. Not only does TendoFit help your tendons work the way they're supposed to... When compared to the control group, **TendoFit promoted a significant improvement in joint comfort, too.**

Now I can already hear the voices of mainstream naysayers yapping on about how these are just two small studies... And how you should wait decades while they conduct their own research and studies and gobble up credit they don't deserve...

But I say hooey! Why wait when Ultimate Tendon Support is available right now. Well you won't have to wait so long as I have something to say about it.

But before I tell you how you can get your hands on Ultimate Tendon Support, I need to tell you about...

The secret supporting ingredient that no one ever thinks of when it comes to tendon health...

You should know I'd never even *think* about putting some "filler" in my formulas. If the two ingredients in TendoFit were enough—we would've stopped right there. And we probably could have.

But as I was about to give Ultimate Tendon Support my stamp of approval, I realized it needed just one more thing. It's an old stand-by but it's *never* been used like this before...

Of course you've heard of vitamin C...

I've spoken often of this superstar vitamin but it's also one of your tendons' greatest allies. Because vitamin C plays a vital role in developing and maintaining the collagen that makes up your tendons, making it an essential nutrient for having strong, healthy tendons.

Plus new preliminary research is starting to crop up showing even more benefits vitamin C could have for your tendons.

For example, in a recent study on animals, one group was given high dose IV vitamin C while the control group received none. And after just 21 days, the results weren't just great—they were downright astounding.

First of all, the vitamin C group **produced more collagen than the control.**

But *even more* incredible, when examined, the vitamin C group also had more new tendon tissue than the control group. **And that was after just 21 days!**

As soon as I confirmed that, I got on the phone right away and said we had to have vitamin C in the formula. And I'm glad we did, because I can't wait to see the full potential of vitamin C unfold as more studies are completed.

As I mentioned, the research for this incredible formula was conducted in Europe. So some lucky folks over there have already had the chance to give it a try.

And from athletes trying to stay in peak condition to regular folks with stressed tendons from everyday life, this supplement has proven itself time and time again.

And now you don't have to wait another minute for this revolutionary formula—Ultimate Tendon Support is now available in the U.S.! (See page 410 for ordering information.)

Chapter 42:

The Real Miracle for Arthritis Pain

The real miracle for joint pain and swelling has been sitting right under our noses for decades in the form of cortisone.

Hold on... I know what you're thinking. Everything you hear and read nowadays tells you that cortisone can ruin your health. And it can, but so can any other substance if it's overused, including water. When cortisone's powers were first discovered, doctors got carried away and gave massive—and often destructive—doses.

Actually, cortisol is a normal hormone and is absolutely essential for life. With this in mind, a doctor by the name of William Jeffries hypothesized that since cortisol occurs naturally in the body, it must be safe in proper physiologic amounts. Jeffries went on to spend years researching the potential benefits of cortisol.

Dr. Jeffries' research found that small, safe dosages of cortisol can be dramatically beneficial in treating chronic fatigue syndrome, rheumatoid arthritis and other autoimmune disorders, and chronic allergic disorders such as hay fever or asthma.

Action to take:

If you have lingering joint pain or anti-immune problems you can't get rid of, consider cortisone treatment.

Cortisol is available only by prescription, and treatment should be closely monitored by a qualified physician.

For a referral to such a physician in your area, please contact the American College for Advancement in Medicine at (800) 532-3688, or online at www.acam.org.

Chapter 43:

Experience the ultimate muscle-pumper that has the fitness freaks crying, "NO FAIR!" Stay STRONG, stand TALL and feel FIT with the help of just one little secret

Let me make one thing clear... the secret you're about to discover does NOT involve sweating till you're soaked. And there's no wallet-zapping memberships or new age body-twisting yoga either.

In fact, with *this secret* <u>you can pump your muscles and feel surging energy and strength</u>. Imagine maintaining your muscles while spending more time in your La-Z-Boy and less time lifting weights. That's the power behind your little secret...

- After one day **you can feel a boost of energy**

- After two weeks **you could be popping open jars and lifting grocery bags with a knowing smile**

- And after just one month **your friends**

and family will be asking, "where do you workout?"

It's high time to leave those torturous treadmills to the fitness freaks and hamsters. You're smarter than that and with this one **superhero nutrient** you can feel stronger, too.

Take the "work" *out* of your work-out. Keeping strong, lean, tight muscles is *so easy!*

What you're about to discover can be *your little secret*. You see, your friends and family will want to know how you're maintaining strong, fit muscles—all without spending hours at the gym.

But they're thinking about muscle maintenance the wrong way! Soaking yourself in sweat is not the only answer. In fact the latest research reveals this amazing secret behind saving muscle strength!

You know how skeptical I am about fitness propaganda. So here's the bottom line: If your muscles are weakening it's not necessarily because you need more exercise! The latest research shows muscle loss is also biological.

Muscle loss happens regardless of your fitness level, even in master athletes like professional baseball players! So you can pound the pavement, row like a water-bug, or pump iron like the former Governor of California if you want. But protecting your ability to golf, fish, even carry the groceries begins not just with exercise, but with maintaining the muscles you've got by giving them the nutrients they need.

The superhero nutrient that makes the difference between having abs or 'flabs'

If you've read anything I've written in the last 25 years you'll know I'm a huge fan of creatine. Your body naturally makes this amino acid and it can also be obtained from sources of protein. It's used to supply energy to your muscle tissues. And this nutrient has been shown to help fuel muscle repair in your biceps and abs, even the muscles of your heart, stomach, and intestines!

Creatine may be your most important muscle-nourishing nutrient!

However, most men over 60 don't make enough creatine to maintain their muscle and strength, much less regain what time has stolen. But now, mounting evidence shows supplemental creatine can in fact help build lean muscle and strength far better than taking nothing at all, by giving your muscles the energy to work longer and harder so you get the most out of your exercise and your life.

Finally, complete muscle-building support all in one place!

Despite the research, the only creatine supplements you are likely to find are formulated for bodybuilder types. And very few "body preeners" do it right. Their creatine only supplements push double, triple, even quadruple creatine doses to stimulate greater muscle mass. It's an exercise in sheer narcissism, not good health. That's why I want to tell you about **Ultimate Bionic Plus**.

It's the first formula I've found that offers concentrated muscle strengthening nutrition in just the right amount. Each serving contains the recommended 2,000 mg of creatine in a delicious drink, plus 6 more muscle invigorating nutrients.

You won't end up looking like an over-muscled iron-pumper, but don't be surprised if you suddenly feel more energized and fit and all you've done is play golf. And imagine the next time you open a jar of pickles, there's no more struggling with the lid, it pops open on the spot. Even carrying the groceries in can seem easier and less tiring.

But creatine is only the beginning...

A morning of fishing, an afternoon of yard work and your muscles are still going strong!

A second amino acid named taurine is also essential for muscle function.

Taurine helps send the signals from your brain to your muscles telling them to move. And this signaling isn't just to the muscles in your arms or legs. It's signaling ALL of your muscles from your biceps and quadriceps to the muscles in your stomach, intestines, bladder— even your heart!

During a test of muscle function in 2004,

scientists found mice that were deficient in taurine were physically inferior as compared to mice with adequate taurine levels. They showed that taurine was crucial for muscle function and total exercise capacity!

Of course, more studies will need to be done to prove exactly how taurine benefits muscle cells. But all of the current research is pointing to one simple fact: Increase your taurine levels and your muscles just plain work better. And who wouldn't want that?

Ultimate Bionic Plus gives you the creatine and the taurine your muscles need!

Put the brakes on 'shrinking' strength with this little-known muscle booster

Betaine does so many good things for your body especially your muscles. For starters it may help improve your energy level and mood, it even supports your heart health...and it can also help improve muscle performance.

Scientists are finding betaine may increase strength and endurance! Recently, two studies were mentioned in an *American Journal of Clinical Nutrition* review article demonstrating greater performance among runners using betaine.

Of course, I'm not recommending you start training for a marathon, but betaine could put a little extra zip in your step. It may also help your body synthesize creatine for even better results.

But despite all of this great news, most men aren't being told about betaine much less how to supplement with it. Which is why I feel really good about giving you a quality dose of muscle-supporting betaine in every serving of Ultimate Bionic Plus.

Plus my formula contains essential mineral support in the right dosage and form to help control muscle cramping!

Everyone gets leg cramps from time to time and when a shooting leg cramp rouses you in the middle of the night there's nothing to do but walk it out. The fitness freaks are quick to scold, "You need to stretch more!" or, "You're not drinking enough water!" But your muscles don't need to be pulled and prodded like Stretch Armstrong or drowned like a fish—what they're likely aching for is good old-fashioned minerals...

IT'S A FACT: Muscle cramps are usually a sign your muscles are overworked and in need of nutrients!

There are many supplements that claim to help leg cramps but I haven't found one with just the right dosage and form your muscles really need! Ultimate Bionic Plus gives you the exact muscle-mending trio of minerals, starting with magnesium...

The magnesium supplements I've seen use the WRONG FORM. Research shows magnesium citrate is the one that can make all of the difference...

During a randomized, crossover placebo controlled trial, 46 patients supplemented with 300 mg magnesium citrate. After 6 weeks 78 percent told Keele University researchers they thought the magnesium helped their legs feel better overall!

You'll get magnesium citrate in every glass of Ultimate Bionic Plus for feel-good muscles! And then there's potassium...

Everyone knows potassium's good for your muscles. Countless studies have linked too little potassium with muscle cramps, including one from the famed Linus Pauling Institute! The research suggests replenishing your levels can not only help relieve and prevent muscle cramps, it even helps prevent muscle fatigue.

Potassium levels decline as you get older, which can lead to feelings of lethargy and weakness. Yet most supplements give you piddly amounts, rarely over 99 mg! That's why I made sure Ultimate Bionic Plus gives you a therapeutic dose of 900 mg of potassium—that's almost 10 times the potassium you'll find in most supplements! And finally, I included...

Calcium plus vitamin D to sustain healthy muscle fibers. One of the most easily absorbed forms of calcium is Calcium Lactate, and that's the form I included in Ultimate Bionic Plus.

But it is not just the ingredients that make Ultimate Bionic Plus different from any other product of its kind...

Ultimate Bionic Plus relies on effervescent

delivery so it is easy to take. All 7 muscle-supporting nutrients dissolve in a glass of water so you know they'll be absorbed into every muscle in your body! Unlike pills, there's no waiting and no waste!

And heck, it's a lot more convenient than working yourself up into a sweat.

While I'm not recommending you lie on the couch all day and watch T.V., you don't have to live at the gym either! It's always a good idea to touch base with your doctor about the exercise and nutrition program that's best for you.

But you can rest assured that with Ultimate Bionic Plus you'll have complete muscle nutrition so your normal activities like a walk around the block, a few holes of golf, even taking out the trash can seem so much easier, you'll have more energy to do the other physical activities you love. All the while you can protect your new-found fitness against age-related loss:

- Just rip open the packet...

- Pour it in a glass of water...

- Watch it fizz up, dissolve and drink up...

You'll send a surge of fortifying nourishment to hungry muscles with every cool and delicious glass.

And you can do it all for LESS THAN HALF of what you'll pay for most gym memberships... (See page 410 for ordering information.)

Chapter 44:

10 More Ways to Make Life More Enjoyable by Just Saying "No" to Junk Medicine

---

#1) Regenerate old brain cells and reverse the effects of brain aging

Acetyl-L-carnitine (ALC) is an amino acid that has been shown to be effective in preventing neuron loss in the brain's memory centers. An Italian study showed that it also boosts a substance in your system called "nerve growth factor" (NGF) that regenerates old neurons and stimulates new ones.

ALC occurs naturally in the brain, but your brain's supply of it diminishes with age. Supplementing your brain's amount of ALC has been shown to not only improve cognitive ability but also to bring about positive structural and neurochemical changes. ALC promotes the release and synthesis of acetylcholine in the brain, something else that degenerates with age because of the decrease in the brain's cholinergic receptors. ALC also takes care of that by restoring those receptors.

Although ALC is found in most high-protein animal foods, it is difficult to obtain therapeutic amounts from your diet alone.

Action to take:

ALC is available in most health-food stores. It should be refrigerated there and once you get it home. Begin a cycle in which you supplement with 1,000 mg of ALC each day for one month, then take a month off, then return to the supplements once again, and so on.

#2) Drink to your health—and to prevent Alzheimer's

A study published by the French medical journal *Revue Neurologique* indicates that moderate consumption of wine (three to four glasses per day) considerably reduces the risk and frequency of senile dementia for those over 65 years of age.

Furthermore, the study states that after three years of monitoring over 3,700 people, researchers found a 75 percent reduction in the incidence of Alzheimer's disease when compared to those abstaining from alcohol.

The number of all senile dementia cases was reduced by 80 percent. (This figure also included the statistics for Alzheimer's disease.)

Action to take:

There is compelling evidence that moderate wine consumption can be relatively benefi-

*cial to overall health. And there is fur-
ther evidence that the reduction of senile
dementia is even greater when the study's
people drank three to four glasses of wine
per day rather than one or two.*

While the evidence from one study isn't enough
for doctors to start prescribing a couple of
alcoholic drinks a day for their patients, it
would seem to me that enjoying a glass of wine
or two or a cold beer with dinner certainly
won't hurt you.

#3) Debunking the calcium myths

Osteoporosis is a serious problem. It af-
fects 10 million Americans (two-thirds of whom
are women). The good news is that you can prevent it with proper nutrition. And young people
would be wise to start early. You can build
and store away bone for old age, much like you
would with money in a retirement bank account.

If you watch TV and read mainstream maga-
zines, you probably believe that all you have
to do to avoid osteoporosis is pop some calcium supplements. This is a good example of
Junk Medicine. And according to a recent study
by Dr. Constance Kies of the University of Ne-
braska, "taking calcium supplements may actually make osteoporosis even worse."

You can take all the calcium in the world,
and it won't do you a lick of good if you're not
getting enough vitamin D (5,000 to 25,000 units
a day) and magnesium (500-1,000 mg).

The truth is, the average person's diet is rarely calcium deficient. The problem with calcium, however, is that many people don't absorb it properly.

In order to properly assimilate calcium, your body must be on the alkaline side. And in order for your body to be on the alkaline side, you have to have enough vitamin D, magnesium, and manganese.

Several studies have shown that laboratory animals that did not get enough manganese had twice the occurrence rates of osteoporosis as animals on a manganese-sufficient diet. And a recent study from Belgium backed up this finding. It found that every person with osteoporosis was manganese-deficient.

Action to take:

You must first find out if you're getting enough vitamin D and, therefore, absorbing enough calcium. You can do this by determining your body's pH level.

Test kits for pH levels, called Hydrion papers or Nitrazine strips, are available in most drug stores. If your pH levels indicate that you are deficient, increase the amount of vitamin D you're taking by 5,000 units.

Also, have a good holistic doctor check your magnesium and manganese levels. For a referral to a holistic physician in your area, contact the American College for Advancement in Medicine at (800) 532-3688.

#4) A health secret of some of the world's most powerful people

What do Winston Churchill, Thomas Edison, Napoleon, and JFK have in common? They were all nappers.

I've been advocating a midday nap my whole working life. It will make you more productive and alert, and will help give your body the proper rest it needs.

For me, 30 minutes to an hour is perfect. As soon as I wake up, I have a cup of coffee. I don't recommend you sleep much more than an hour. If you do, you may find it hard to go to sleep at night.

Action to take:

Try taking a 30-minute to one-hour nap every day this week. I think you'll be surprised how good it makes you feel. For more information, check out The Art of Napping, a book by William Anthony.

#5) Iron: Too much of a good thing could kill you

When most people think about iron, they worry about not getting enough. But really, only about 1 percent of the adult population suffers from iron deficiency (anemia).

Most older Americans get more iron than they need. Since high levels of iron are linked to increases in heart disease, diabetes, and cancer, this is certainly something to be concerned about.

Dr. Richard Wood of the Center on Aging at Tufts University said, "We found that about 91 percent of the population we looked at had dietary iron intakes that were greater than the recommended dietary levels."

Meat, fish, eggs, and whole grains have heavy concentrations of iron. But the problem isn't with eating a lot of meat. The real problem is that food manufacturers have gone ahead and enriched so many of the products they put on the market with iron. This is great for that one percent of anemic people, but for the rest of us it could do more harm than good.

Actions to take:

Avoid extra iron in your diet. You can eat all the meat you want, but cut back on processed foods. If you eat a lot of meat, be careful with dosage amounts of vitamin C, which makes you absorb iron. Also, stop taking vitamins and supplements that contain iron.

Second, have your doctor run a serum ferritin determination. If your test levels are high, donate a pint of blood; that should bring your body's store of iron back to normal.

Finally, drink some coffee. The anti-coffee freaks of the Junk Medicine world have tried to convince us that coffee is bad. In fact, quite the opposite is true. Cof-

fee is good for you for several reasons, one of which is the fact that it will help protect you from iron overload.

#6) The soy ploy—what you need to know about this meat substitute

According to some popular media myths, soybean products are the answer to good health. Soy, they say, provides high quality protein, while cutting your risk of heart disease, protecting you against cancer, and relieving symptoms for menopausal woman.

Guess what—not a single one of these points has been medically proven.

Soy products will lower your cholesterol levels, but they WILL NOT cut your risk of heart disease. As I explained in Chapter 3, low cholesterol levels do not protect you from heart problems. Just the opposite, in fact: Low cholesterol may indeed cause heart problems and strokes.

Second, soy does not protect you from cancer. A study by the British government in 1997 found that the only place soy or soy-related products inhibit cancer growth is in test tubes.

As for menopausal symptoms, placebos have been proven to be just as effective.

Action to take:

Do not eschew meat for soy and think it's going to help you be healthy. Soy definitely causes more problems than it will prevent. And I don't know about you, but I think the stuff tastes rotten.

My advice? Take it easy on soy products. Having it occasionally probably won't hurt you, but don't give up things like eggs, butter, cream, beef, pork, fish, chicken, and lamb to do it.

Also, keep in mind that when you take soy products, you'll certainly need to up your levels of vitamin B12.

Plus, an element of soy called d. phytic acid will block your body's absorption of important nutrients,such as calcium, magnesium, iron, and zinc—so be sure to increase your doses of those as well if you consume anything containing soy.

#7) CPR can be either a killer or a lifesaver—how to do it properly

You've seen it on TV dramas. Medics rush to give a drowning victim CPR…but the patient still dies.

Unfortunately, this is more than just a TV story line. It's happening in real life, because too many people are following the classic CPR taught in outdated textbooks. As a result, CPR is killing the very people it was meant to save. This is especially true in drowning situations and in severe asthma attacks.

CPR is for heart attacks, not asthma attack or drowning victims. Asthma sufferers experi-

ence an increase in mucous production during
an attack. This mucous forms a plug that blocks
the airways, preventing air from reaching the
lungs. Drowning victims have swallowed water,
which causes blockage to their lungs. In both
situations, performing classic CPR actually
forces the obstruction even deeper.

The first step should be to dislodge the obstruction using the Heimlich maneuver.

Actions to take:

When the victim is lying on the ground:

1. *Place the victim on his back. Turn his
   face to one side to allow water to drain
   from his mouth.*

2. *Facing the victim, kneel astride his
   hips.*

3. *With one of your hands on top of the
   other, place the heel of your bottom
   hand on the upper abdomen below the rib
   cage and above the navel.*

4. *Use your body weight to press into the
   victim's upper abdomen with a quick upward thrust.*

*Repeat until water no longer flows from the
mouth or mucous is dispelled.*

If the victim is standing:

1. *Stand behind the victim and wrap your
   arms around his waist.*

2. *Make a fist and place the thumb side of your fist against the victim's upper abdomen, below the rib cage and above the navel.*

3. *Grasp your fist with your other hand and press into the victim's upper abdomen with a quick upward thrust. Do not squeeze the rib cage; confine the force of the thrust to your hands.*

4. *Repeat until water no longer flows from the mouth or mucous is dispelled.*

After performing one of the above techniques, if the victim has not recovered, you can then perform traditional CPR. Be sure to get the victim to a doctor as quickly as possible.

#8) Drug-free ways to boost your energy levels

These days, mainstream treatment for low energy levels seems to be centered on selective serotonin-reuptake inhibitors or SSRIs. It can be easy to take a prescription from your doctor and mask your symptoms, but it's important to note that SSRIs do nothing to address the underlying cause of energy loss.

The first thing you must realize is that the lack of energy is not your problem but rather a symptom of your problem. To fix it, you first must determine what your underlying problem is… then you can take steps to cure it.

Actions to take:

*If you're experiencing low energy lev-
els, start by getting some daily exercise.
Nothing too strenuous—perhaps a 30-minute
walk. Lifting light weights is also good.*

*Next, if you're not sleeping well, get
your melatonin levels checked, and if they
are low, start taking this hormone.*

*If a lack of sleep is not your problem, try
the following vitamins and herbs:*

*Vitamin B12: This vitamin is vital to every
person's health, young or old, and is the
first thing a doctor should recommend for low
energy levels. It's usually administered in
the form of injections, because some people
have a hard time absorbing it. However, oral
supplements are also worth trying. Be sure
you get at least 250 mcg a day. Meat is the
best natural source of B12.*

*One thing to note: If you are taking large
amounts of vitamin C (1,200 mg or more),
you may have a hard time absorbing the
B12 your body needs. So if your energy
levels are low and you are taking large
amounts of vitamin C, cut back your vitamin C intake to absorb more vitamin B12.
It can also help to take your vitamin C
pill and your B12 pill at different times
of the day.*

*Ginger: You can get ginger naturally or
in supplement form. For supplements, take*

100 mg of ginger root powder daily if your energy levels are low.

Ginseng: You'll find many varieties of ginseng, but the two most worth trying are Siberian and Panax. Ginseng has a cumulative effect, so you have to take it for several weeks before you'll notice a difference. I recommend 75 mg of a high-quality Panax ginseng or 150 mg of Siberian ginseng.

Gotu kola: Think of this herb as caffeine, without the side effects. You can use it much like you would ginger (but it doesn't taste as good). I recommend 50 mg of gotu kola per day.

#9) Health scam revealed: Don't waste your money on "vitamin O"

There is a new trend of taking drops of "liquid oxygen," which are being marketed as the fictional nutrient "vitamin O."

The idea of taking oxygen by drops is ludicrous. The lungs are designed for the absorption of oxygen. The gastrointestinal tract is designed to absorb food. Attempting to eat oxygen is about as ridiculous as trying to breathe food.

#10) Exercise that prolongs your life— without even making you break a sweat

Strenuous physical activity is guaranteed by health "experts" to give you a longer life. Your tissues need oxygen to stay healthy (and to keep you feeling young). The theory is that if you exercise vigorously, you will increase the oxygenation of the blood and, in turn, your tissues.

This is simply not true. In fact, the harder you exercise, the lower the oxygen content in your blood, since the body burns oxygen to cover the work load. When your cells don't get enough oxygen, they degenerate and die.

Eventually, this causes YOU to degenerate and die.

There is a way to get the anti-aging, super-longevity effects of exercise you've heard about—it's a method called EWOT, which stands for Exercise with Oxygen Therapy.

Exercising while breathing bottled oxygen dramatically increases the amount of oxygen in the blood plasma. This extra plasma-oxygen results in an extensive increase in your total tissue-oxygen level. And the best part? You need only about 15 minutes of mild to moderate exercise with oxygen per day to achieve these anti-aging effects!

Putting EWOT into practice couldn't be easier. The hardest part will be obtaining the bottle of oxygen necessary to carry out the exercise. In most states, oxygen is available only by prescription. For a referral to an alternative physician who will be open to this treatment, contact ACAM at (800)532-3688 or www.acam.org. Once you've got the oxygen bottle and are ready to begin exercise (whatever form you choose—from walking on a treadmill, to riding

a stationary bike, to simply lifting light bar-
bells), set the oxygen flow to 6 liters per minute, attach the nasal oxygen tube, and begin.
After 15 minutes of EWOT, there is a dramatic
"pinking up" of the skin. This means that even
the tiny capillaries are carrying oxygen to
your body's cells. In essence, if you're pink
and you feel better, it's working! This method
of prolonging your life is so simple that it's
hard to believe it could work—but it does, and
you can do it without even breaking a sweat!

Chapter 45:

Big Pharma Hopes You Never Find Out About This Ayurvedic Herb That Puts Alzheimer's Drugs to Shame

Since the first time your wife forgot where she was going, you started worrying that it might be Alzheimer's disease. And as it becomes more usual for her to forget things—like your grandson's name—your worry is getting bigger and bigger.

The possibility is like a knife to your gut. And thinking about nursing homes and pharmaceuticals does nothing to ease that fear.

Even if it's not the total devastation of Alzheimer's disease, memory loss and slower, muddled thinking can have a very negative impact on both of your lives.

And you're right to want to face that head on... slow it down, even revive some of that fading memory... but you're also right to not trust the pharmaceuticals your doctor will probably recommend. You won't find the answer in mainstream medicine. But you will find it here.

The answer is an ancient, time-tested Ayurvedic herb. Its safety has been proven by generations of use. And its effectiveness has been proven in numerous scientific studies.

This is not a pill cooked up to line a Big Pharma executive's pockets at the expense of your loved ones. This is a real solution to memory, concentration, and cognition problems. It won't hurt the people you love, and it won't cost your retirement savings. It will help restore brain power, and may even keep the full devastation of Alzheimer's disease at bay.

Powerful herb protects and improves your precious brain power

For centuries, this Ayurvedic herb has been used to protect and boost the mind, intellect and consciousness.

This small creeping herb can be spotted throughout northeastern India, in the marshy areas alongside ponds and streams. Known as *Brahmi* in Ayurveda, bacopa monniera impacts your brain in many positive ways.

In addition to enhancing cognitive abilities, bacopa also helps ease anxiety and agitation (it's actually used traditionally to treat psychosis), increases the amount of new information your brain can retain, and combats mental fatigue.

Even more telling, in Ayurveda bacopa is

used to prevent, treat, and fight dementia, even Alzheimer's disease. That traditional use is now being backed up by solid science, with more human clinical trials in progress as this is being written.

Unlike the pharmaceuticals doctors prescribe for Alzheimer's, bacopa comes with no contraindications, and no severe—or deadly—side effects.

The best thing about Alzheimer's drugs is that they don't work

Not working sounds like a bad thing, and it is. But, honestly, compared to the truly devastating damage the pharmaceuticals (like Aricept and Exelon) designed to treat desperate Alzheimer's patients can do, simply not working is better.

The drug companies prey on your fear, guilt, and hope. And they don't even bother to pretend that their drugs really work, or that they don't cause terrible side effects. In fact, all you have to do is look at the Aricept website to see a long list of common side effects—not the worst ones, just the most common. Here are a few that strike so many patients they're prominently posted on the home page:

- Slow heartbeat

- Fainting

- Difficulty sleeping

- Difficulty passing urine

- Seizures

- Increased stomach acid

- Diarrhea

- Vomiting

- Feeling tired

- Muscle cramps

- Loss of appetite

- Worsening lung problems (like asthma)

So the drugs don't work in any meaningful way. And they cause horrible side effects. And the fact that they are FDA-approved underlines just how little you can trust the agency to protect you.

To be perfectly clear: Please stay away from these dangerous drugs.

Because there is something better, safer, and effective that may truly help your loved ones hold on to their precious brain power, and maybe even regain some function you feared was lost.

Studies show that Bacopa helps where pharmaceuticals fail

Some of the earliest signs of Alzheimer's disease are easily taken for normal signs of aging. Because slowing down, forgetting where your keys are, taking longer to remember your neighbor's dog's name... that happens to everyone.

But whether or not it's due to that over-whelming disease, you don't have to accept it. You can improve your memory, sharpen your mind, increase new learning, boost concentration, and even calm nervous anxiety with a very safe, very effective ancient herb, bacopa.

Rigorous study has found that this herb especially impacts how your brain handles new information: Bacopa is proven to help you retain more of it.

- A 2002 double-blind, randomized, placebo-controlled study[1] found a significant impact of bacopa "for the retention of new information." Researchers also noted that bacopa slowed down how quickly subjects forgot new information.

- A more recent randomized, double-blind, placebo-controlled study[2] of 81 subjects (all at least 55 years old) showed that bacopa significantly improved "memory acquisition and retention."

- In a 2008 study[3] subjects taking bacopa every day for 90 days saw significantly improved accuracy for their spatial working memory (critical for being able to find things and remember where they are).

Bacopa helps cognition and memory in so many ways, but just as important is its impact on your peace of mind.

Peace of mind and a sense of calm

Agitation... irritability... anxiety... they strike all of us now and then, and some of us more often than not. Which brings us to bacopa's other positive power: It helps bring on a sense of calm and clarity of mind.

In fact, that soothing ability is so strong that it even helps in cases of severe mental illness, like schizophrenia. A 2012 case study[4] found that adding 500 mg per day of bacopa to standard treatments for schizophrenia helped control symptoms more than the standard alone, without adverse effects.

And when it comes to anxiety, bacopa can really help calm things down. A brand new study[5], published just as this article is being written, found that 450 mg of bacopa daily for four weeks helped ease anxiety better than placebo.

Now, short-term memory issues and increasing anxiety are two very common symptoms that plague Alzheimer's patients. But can bacopa really help them fight this devastating disease?

Real, safe help for Alzheimer's patients

Though there hasn't yet been a clinical study investigating the impact of bacopa on Alzheimer's disease, many researchers believe that this Ayurvedic herb could offer a world of protection. And they're backing that up with the beginnings of some very substantial research.

One clinical study[6] of healthy individuals determined that one important way bacopa helps improve cognition, attention, and working memory is by suppressing a brain chemical known as AChE (acetylcholinesterase). If that chemical rings a bell—it should. AChE is a key target of most existing Alzheimer's drugs, the class known as cholinesterase inhibitors that includes Razadyne, Exelon, and Aricept. Bacopa seems to hit that same target, without bringing on intolerable side effects.

And an exciting new lab study[7] found that bacopa could be a very powerful ally in the fight against Alzheimer's disease. It turns out that one way bacopa protects your brain and improves memory is by increasing the activity of an enzyme known as the sodium-potassium pump. That enzyme seems to play a very important role in brain cells and brain health, and could shine a light on a whole new tactic for fighting Alzheimer's disease.

And though this animal study was conducted before the one you just read about, it also found a positive impact on the sodium-potassium pump enzyme. For this study,[8] scientists use an animal model of dementia to see just how much protection bacopa could offer. After treatment with bacopa, memory impairment was reversed, and oxidative damage was repaired. In addition, the bacopa restored sodium-potassium pump action in the treated rats. The researchers conclusion: "The results suggest therapeutic potential of bacopa monnieri in the treatment of AD [Alzheimer's disease] associated cognitive decline."

Finally, researchers conducting another animal study[9] reported that bacopa "is a potential cognitive enhancer and neuroprotectant against Alzheimer's disease."

Which bacopa can you trust?

With more interest in bacopa, you can expect some less than reputable sources to spring up. And when you're dealing with something as precious as your mind, you want to make sure your herbs come from someone deserving your trust.

The research team Himalaya Herbal Healthcare showed me not one, but two clinical trials on their bacopa. And the results were very much in line with the many published studies we've talked about.

The first study included 100 subjects, all with some symptoms of memory, learning or concentration distur-bance. During the four-week trial, subjects took either one bacopa caplet or placebo daily. And by the end of the trial, the bacopa group experienced some substantial results:

- 75 percent had reduced irritability

- 66 percent had a resurgence in energy

- More than 50 percent were less tired

- 80 percent had improved memory

- 36 percent had improved concentration

- 37 percent increased learning ability

With such positive results from their first

trial, the company ran a second clinical trial. In this study, 50 volunteers with cognitive disturbances took one bacopa caplet every day for twelve weeks. And there were improvements in every measure: visual reaction time, verbal reasoning, working memory, and logical memory. The researchers noted that this success might be partly due to the special chemicals (triterpenide saponins and bacosides) in the herb that improve brain cell communication.

And in addition to the successful brain boost, no adverse events were reported or observed during either of the trials, making Himalaya Herbal Bacopa a safe, effective choice.

Boost your brain power and fight Alzheimer's disease with Bacopa

There is a safe, effective, real solution for diminishing brain power, whether it's from the normal impact of aging or something much more serious like Alzheimer's diseases. Bacopa delivers what drug companies wish that they could, a way to meaningfully improve memory and focus... without subjecting you to dangerous, even deadly, side effects.

The manufacturer recommends taking one caplet of Bacopa every day on an empty stomach.

You can find ordering information for Bacopa in your Wellness Directory on page 409.

Chapter 46:

How to Survive Your Surgery

"Never" sure isn't what it used to be, folks—because the worst-of-the-worst surgical mistakes that are "never" supposed to happen keep right on happening with shocking frequency.

Imagine going in for an operation on your right arm... and waking up to find the doc performed the procedure on your left instead.

Well, this week alone, 20 people don't have to imagine it—because it happened to them (let's hope they weren't amputations). Another 20 patients had surgery on the right spot, but got the wrong operation, according to damning new numbers from a Johns Hopkins University study.

And 39 times every week, a doctor accidentally leaves something inside a patient—like a piece of surgical equipment (or, who knows, maybe his graduation ring).

It adds up to 4,000 surgical "never" events every year—and if the doctor thinks he can get away with it, he won't even tell you that he's botched the job. All you know is you're suddenly setting off metal detectors everywhere you go.

And that's if you're lucky. As you can imagine, most of the victims of botched surgery find out the hard way: They're hurt... sometimes badly, with 40 percent suffering permanent injury and 6.6 percent of them killed by mistakes that "never" should have happened in the first place.

And those are just the ones we know of. Trust me, hospitals are even better than politicians at covering up their mistakes.

The number of "never" mistakes during surgery is already inexcusable—but they represent just a small part of the picture. Medical mistakes in general KILL close to 100,000 Americans every year—and hundreds of thousands of others are injured, often badly, by their so-called care.

That's such a miserable track record that if medical screw-ups were a disease, it would be the...

Fifth leading cause of death in the nation!

That's right. As a "disease," medical mistakes would rank behind only heart disease, cancer, lower respiratory disease, and stroke. It would be deadlier than diabetes and twice as deadly as pneumonia and flu—and that's assuming you believe the inflated "official" flu numbers (I sure as heck don't).

There's no vaccine against stupidity and no drug that will protect you from carelessness, so you need to rely on the most natural and time-honored cure of all: Yourself.

You need to remain vigilant and watch your doctors and nurses like a hawk. The catch-22, of course, is that you can't always do that when you're in a hospital—and you certainly can't keep an eye on a darned thing once they put you under for surgery.

So follow these steps and get the whole family in on the act:

Hold a family meeting: This will be about as much fun as a timeshare presentation, and without the promise of a free night's stay in a luxury resort. But it's necessary—because everyone in the family needs to be able to keep an eye out for everyone else if an emergency lands someone in the hospital.

Appoint a historian: Everyone in the family—especially the seniors—should have a "historian." Your historian should be someone who can come with you to doctor and keep a notebook of what you're told, especially if you're preparing for surgery. Even if you're sharp as a tack—and, if you're a *Douglass Report* reader, I'm sure you are—preparing for surgery can be overwhelming and confusing. Your historian will help you sort through it all, and can also ask the questions when you can't.

Invest in a magic marker: If you're going under anesthesia, write notes all over your body beforehand. Turn yourself into the illustrated man (or woman) with phrases like "NOT

HERE" and "WRONG ARM" along with an "X" to mark the spot to help make sure you don't wake up with any surprises.

Meet your doctor: Ask to speak to the surgeon right before surgery, and don't let them start the anesthesia until you do. Tell him you have a last minute question. The question itself doesn't matter, the real goal is to make sure the doc knows who you are, what procedure he's doing, and where. If he starts to look puzzled or surprised at any point, get out of that room as quickly as you can.

The sad reality is that medical incompetence is like incompetence anywhere else—if there's a way to screw something up, you can bet someone will find it. So there's no surefire way to make sure you won't be a victim of a medical mistake, "never" or otherwise.

But with careful action, thorough planning and a vigilant family standing by your side, you can minimize your risk.

Chapter 47:

Have You Been a Guinea Pig for the Latest, "Greatest" Surgical Scams? Read This Before You Go Under the Knife!

How does it feel to be a guinea pig? You say you don't know? Well, if you've ever had surgery, there's a good chance you were a big old human guinea pig. See, most people don't know that new surgical procedures really are new. That is, they have not been investigated for efficacy or safety. Can you imagine what would happen if a doctor did this with a natural supplement or therapy (like, oh, I don't know... photoluminescence)? They'd pack him off to the pokey for 20 years. It seems that white-collar crime, or white-coat crime, is now more severely punished than rape or murder. But surgeons are different. They can do pretty much whatever they please. They just "invent" a surgical procedure and keep doing it until someone finally tests it scientifically to see if it really works. And the real kicker is that these procedures are often proven to be completely bogus when patients in the placebo group fare as well as those actually getting the surgery.

That's right—that "dramatic improvement" from an operation can be entirely delusional. In surgical studies, sometimes the patient wakes up from anesthesia symptom-free—completely cured—when the surgeon has done nothing but make a superficial incision then sew it up.

Mind over medical procedure: Placebo surgery produces the same— and sometimes __better__—results than the "real thing"

One of the biggest surgical scams going on these days is arthroscopic surgery for arthritis of the knee. Don't get me wrong; this type of surgery for knee __injuries__ is nothing short of miraculous: Football players who tear their knee ligaments can usually return to full duty in a matter of weeks with this surgery. But some orthopedist with dollar signs in his eyes got the bright idea that if arthroscopic surgery was good for knee injuries, why not try it out on arthritic knees? Maybe you could diddle around in the joint space, doing a cleanup of whatever trash you could find in there, and, presto, no more arthritis.

It seemed to work dramatically well for Tim Perez. He had such severe arthritis pain in his knee, he'd resorted to using a cane to help him walk. So when he heard about a study going on at the VA Medical Center in Houston, Texas, that was going to test arthroscopic surgery procedure for knee arthritis, he enrolled, hoping for some much-needed relief. Although it was widely used, the surgery had never been tested for efficacy up until this point. But with the results Mr. Perez experienced, who could doubt the effectiveness of the procedure? After three months, he was pain-free and able to throw away his cane. Two years later, he found out that he'd been in the placebo group of the study—the surgeons hadn't done anything definitive to his knee.

The official results of the study revealed that, like Tim Perez, the majority of the patients who went through the dummy surgery fared as well in perceived knee function and pain reduction as those who had real arthroscopic procedures. In fact, in some cases patients who got the placebo procedure reported <u>better results</u> than some of the actual surgery patients. And after examining their knee structure, researchers reported that neither group showed any measurable improvement in actual (not perceived) knee function. So, basically, this study is saying that arthroscopic surgery for arthritis is pure bunk... but you can bet surgeons are still going to recommend it and perform it. Why?

The endless profit potential of "voodoo surgery"

Well, 650,000 patients each year undergo arthroscopic surgery for arthritic knees, at a cost of $5,000 each. That's over <u>$3 billion</u>— and insurers routinely reimburse for it. This is only one of many surgical procedures that gobble up billions of dollars in insurance payments yearly with <u>no proof of efficacy</u>. *The Wall Street Journal* research department uncovered the following medical "profit centers" that may be useless and, in some cases, harmful:

Spinal fusion—no proof of effectiveness

Thymectomy (excision of the thymus gland in the chest for various diseases)—no proof of effectiveness

Arthroscopic shoulder procedure—no proof of effectiveness

Circumcision—not medically necessary

Action to take:

So is arthroscopic surgery worth it? Tim Perez thinks so. But as for you, I suggest that you stay away from voodoo surgery. That means you should assume all new procedures are voodoo until proven otherwise. If you have arthritis, try one of the following alternatives before giving the surgeon the green light to come at you with a scalpel:

(1) Glucosamine/chondroitin capsules— they're available just about everywhere, and you really can't take too much (within reason, of course). Just follow the dosage instructions on the bottle of the brand you choose.

(2) Devil's claw supplements—this herb is available from health food stores and

even some pharmacies. Take 2 grams a day. While no major side effects appear to be associated with devil's claw, it may interfere with the action of blood thinning drugs like Coumadin; if you are currently taking such medications, you should not begin treatment with devil's claw.

Chapter 48:

Untested... Unregulated... and Unsafe!
THE REAL DIRT ON THE 'CLEAN' CHEMICAL

It's the secret poison millions of Americans **deliberately** rub into their skin every day, several times a day—and most of them have no clue it's even a poison at all.

Heck, most of them believe this chemical junk is actually PROTECTING them—and they go out of their way to use it.

It's a pesticide called triclosan, and don't rest easy if you've never heard the name.

Most people haven't.

But you've definitely heard of antibacterial soap—and that's where you'll find this junk, because triclosan is what gives those suds their supposed super germ-fighting powers.

That's actually just another big, fat lie— because triclosan-laced soap is no better than normal soap. And even if you ditch the antibacterial soap, you still can't leave the triclosan behind, because...

It's absolutely everywhere!

It's the secret ingredient in hand sanitizers, clothing, toothpaste, mouthwash, baby wipes, toys, kitchen utensils, and more. We're exposed to it from every possible direction—so much so that the CDC says this chemical is **_inside 75 percent of us right now_**.

And it's not just casually hanging out in your bloodstream. It's partying like a rock star in a cheap hotel—and you're the hotel, with every single room getting trashed.

That's because this chemical has an all-access pass to your body. It's easily absorbed by cell membranes, including skin cells, and it can get inside anytime you touch it—like when you suds up.

And once inside, it can travel anywhere and everywhere.

It can even travel across the blood-brain barrier.

That means there's no part of your body that triclosan can't wreck—and no end to the damage it can do.

Here's the short list:

BRAIN DAMAGE: Studies on fish and mice have found that triclosan blocks signals between the brain and muscle. The mice had weaker grips (don't ask me how you test that in a mouse, but they did), while fish swam slower in triclosan-laced waters. On the other hand, those fish probably got off lucky since other studies have shown that triclosan in the water can flat-out kill them. And in pregnant women, triclosan could harm the development of the baby's brain.

HEART PROBLEMS: So we know triclosan can disrupt communication between brain and muscle. And in that mice study I just mentioned, it was shown to block signals from the brain to some of the most important muscles of all: the ones that power your heart. Triclosan can actually reduce heart function by as much as 25 percent, according to the study.

SEXUAL DYSFUNCTION: Triclosan is an endocrine disruptor that can screw with thyroid, estrogen, and testosterone. As a result, it's been linked to everything from adult sexual problems such as infertility and low sperm counts to developmental problems in children such as early puberty.

If that's not enough, triclosan can also destroy skin cells, breed superbugs, and may even cause cancer.

Now, I know what you're probably thinking. If this stuff is so bad, why haven't I heard of it? Why is it even allowed in so many products?

Short answer: It ISN'T!

Not technically, anyway. The FDA has never recognized triclosan as safe or effective, and the chemical was even on the verge of being banned decades ago—and then... well... Washington happened.

356 • THE FREE MAN'S DECLARATION FOR HEALTH AND LONGEVITY

A BRIEF HISTORY OF INCOMPETENCE

Back in 1972, Congress ordered the FDA to rule on the safety of a number of chemicals, including triclosan.

Now, you know the FDA. The only reason the agency hasn't written the book on inaction is because that in itself would require action. So the agency was actually acting with lightning speed—for them—when it took a full SIX YEARS to determine there's no evidence triclosan is safe or effective.

As you may have guessed, that's not the end of the story. That's just the beginning—because the FDA never finalized that decision on triclosan, putting it into a sort of limbo where it's not recognized as safe or effective, but not banned either.

And that means more than 40 years after Congress ordered the FDA to rule on triclosan...35 years after the agency decided there was nothing to prove it's safe or effective... companies are still allowed to dump it into practically everything.

In 2012, the FDA said it would finally issue its ruling by December. Except it didn't. Then, the agency said it would issue its rules in February of this year.

Do I even need to tell you what didn't happen in February?

There's talk that ruling could come any day

now. Who knows, it might even happen by the time you read this. But any action they take now will be much too little—and it comes far too late.

And that means it's up to you to protect yourself. (So what else is new?)

Start by avoiding anything with triclosan in it. That's not easy, since it's practically everywhere, and it's not always listed on the label or even advertised. In general, if a product is "antibacterial" or "antimicrobial," then assume there's triclosan in the picture somewhere unless you know otherwise.

Next, arm yourself against bacteria without the help of toxic chemicals. And believe it or not, this is the easy part.

Just follow my...

THREE STEPS FOR SAFE ANTIBACTERIAL PROTECTION

Soap and water: Yes, friends, nothing beats the tried-and-true—and when it comes to keeping clean, nothing's more tried or true than plain old soap and warm water. Dozens of studies have proven that ordinary soap is every bit as effective as antibacterial soap at wiping out germs, and even the feds have admitted as much.

The key isn't to splash and dash. Make sure you really wash your paws by working the soap into your hands for a good 20-30 seconds before rinsing.

Natural immunity: The best offense is a good defense. Boost your own defenses by giving your immune system the power it needs to kill any bacteria that do make it inside. Start with the first few letters of the alphabet—vitamins A, C, and D are all natural immune-boosters. In addition, give your gut the best weapon around against nasty germs: a belly full of GOOD bacteria. That means it's time to take a quality probiotic supplement if you're not on one already.

Common sense: How many people hold onto the escalator handrails in the mall, head up the food court and immediately sit down and eat a burger? If the awful food doesn't do you in, the germs from the unwashed masses all over the escalator railing sure will. So use a little common sense when you're out and about—if you can't avoid contact with germy surfaces such as railings, doorknobs and elevator buttons, then be sure to wash up before you touch food or even rub your eyes.

As I said, this is easy stuff.

In addition, make sure you keep the hard surfaces of your home clean, and that means more than an occasional good scrub. Along with normal soap, feel free to call in the big guns and use a little bleach—especially if someone in your home has been ill or in and out of a care facility such as a hospital or nursing home.

Pay special attention to the kitchen, bathroom, and dining table.

Finally, install a reverse osmosis water filter.

Triclosan is so prevalent that it's even invaded the water supply. It doesn't always reach your tap, but not because your water is clean. It doesn't reach your tap because the water treatment process can cause it to break down and form chemicals that may actually be worse— such as dioxin and chloroform.

You don't want to drink water laced with this stuff. You don't even want to bathe in it—so don't just get that filter, be sure to install it where the water supply enters your home so every sink and tap is covered.

Chapter 49:

The REAL Secrets to a Long Life

Join a gym... eat your veggies... see a therapist... take your meds... The mainstream is just FULL of naggy advice on how to live longer. And isn't it convenient how most of these tips end in a sales pitch?

But you don't have to waste your time OR your money on any of that nonsense. None of it will extend your life. But a recent study that's been 90 years in the making has uncovered the REAL secrets to healthy aging.

And if you've been a reader of mine for any length of time, you already got the inside scoop on these secrets.

Heck, a summary of all 272 pages of "The Longevity Project" reads like a summary of my Douglass Report archives:

- Exercise won't help you to live longer

- You don't have to eat your vegetables

- Stress and worry can be good for you

- Being too optimistic can kill you

Best of all, it's backed by some rock-solid data. The study tracked 1,528 Californians for almost their entire lives, starting in 1921. It went on for so long that the researcher who started it, Lewis Terman, died more than half a century ago!

Fortunately, generations of researchers have continued the project. And the latest team has concluded that...

"Many common health recommendations are ill-advised or simply wrong"

They say steady daily movement like gardening, walking your dog, and even visiting museums is more likely to lead to a longer life than an endless series of exercise failures.

The researchers also found that people who worry and suffer some stress—the creative stress that keeps you focused and driven—live longer than the carefree types we're supposed to envy.

Even marriage doesn't matter as much as most people assume. Married men in the study lived longer than single men and divorcees... but divorced women lived nearly as long as married ones.

Men, you might not like hearing this—but it looks like you need her more than she needs you! I'd tell you not to worry about it... but maybe you should. After all, a little worry is a good thing.

Chapter 50:

Live to 100... Why Stop There?

I'm not saying those bloated, puffed-up pills are bad for you. They may be helping you—a *little*. But I am saying you can do better—much better. **For half the price!**

In my decades of practicing medicine, I've only found four age-busting secrets that pass my toughest tests.

What do I look for in a true anti-aging MVP? It has to make you FEEL FANTASTIC. It has to make you feel STRONG and CHARGED, with your senses firing on all cylinders.

You will never find this kind of exhilarating youth power by applying ointments and creams or scarfing down bowls of cardboard fiber. To me, an anti-aging miracle must...

- Give your heart support that lets you work hard, play hard and enjoy your favorite healthy meals with confidence...

- Make a difference you can feel with energy that keeps you soaring through your favorite activities...

- Support healthy blood pressure, sharp vision, free-moving joints and brain-power that'll keep you outsmarting your friends, kids and grandkids...

And I expect a true youth-pumping hero to do all of the above—and more! Am I setting the bar too high? YOU BET I AM. Get back that youthful feeling with the "POWER 4."

One could help keep your brain snappin' and your heart strong—and you'll never guess how lobsters fit into it all...

Another is getting A LOT of attention these days... and for good reason—the studies on this vitamin will make your head spin!

The third is such powerful support for your joints, heart, brain, skin and so much more— that your friends will be scratching their heads asking, *why can't we feel results like this?*

And the final breakthrough of the "*Power 4*" hails from the other side of world. I'm honored to be one of the first to bring the secret to India's longevity straight to your door.

And today I am bringing the "*Power 4*" to-gether for the first time, in one place with my all you need formula *Ultra Vital Gold*.

This breakthrough "meeting of the miracles" means you have the power to beat back *the most ruthless tricks aging can throw at you.*

The first step is to easily...

Keep your ticker a heart of steel with... Lobsters and Curry?

When did you start giving a hoot how much cholesterol was in your steak and eggs? When was the first time you looked at a heavy box and thought maybe *someone else should lift this...*

It makes sense—the older you get, the more you worry about keeping your heart healthy. So give your heart the support it needs with two heart heroes for ironclad confidence. Your heart was built to last—but just like that truck you've had for decades—*it can benefit from some upkeep.*

Luckily, the mighty maintenance I want to show you doesn't involve a "heave and ho" gym routine. You don't even need to eat a bowl of "shredded cardboard" every morning.

No, to get the kind of support that has been shown in animal studies to:

- Have unbeatable overall heart health benefits...

- Protect against wear and tear caused by exercise...

- And keep blood pressure healthy...

You need unrivaled power that won't bankrupt your piggy bank! How is that possible? It all starts by... Following the lobster's lead... It turns out lobsters have been eating the greatest heart hero for millions of years. The first of the "Power 4" is hiding along the ocean floor in tiny micro algae that lobsters love to munch on. But this is much more than ordinary lobster chow. Its benefits for your heart health (and, as you'll see, entire body) are massive. Like I said, it's so powerful I call it... the Alpha Antioxidant.

It has up to 500 TIMES the antioxidant power of vitamin E! It could help your body promote a healthy inflammatory response. And *lobsters* have been chomping up this heart hero for millions of years?

The proof is in every lobster that's ever graced your dinner plate. Like me, you might have assumed that lobsters turn red in the pot just because of the heat.

It turns out it's not *just* the heat. All their lives, lobsters chow down on the greatest antioxidant God ever created, the deep red Alpha Antioxidant. Lobsters in the wild have a greenish-brown color. But all of their lives they chow down on the Alpha Antioxidant—dying a slight reddish tinge into their shells. So when faced with the 212 degree heat of the boiling water, another protein in the lobster's shell breaks down—and the remaining Alpha Antioxidant red bursts out. If it's powerful enough to stand up to the extreme heat, just imagine what it can do for your heart... The same thing goes for crabs, salmon and shrimp—they're in on the secret, too. So what's so special about it? It makes it so you could... Enjoy life, knowing your heart has breakthrough support!

The Alpha Antioxidant is "hot off the press-es" new—so most of the research comes from animal studies... but these results are too remarkable for you to have to wait any longer.

But with just a few years in the research labs, this heart hero has shown incredible potential and there's no telling what it could do for you...

A 2003 study in mice showed it protected against wear and tear caused by exercise. In a 2006 animal study, it helped maintain healthy blood pressure levels!

And imagine this—in 2005, another animal study revealed the Alpha Antioxidant helped protect and support overall heart health. Remember, this is Mother Nature at her most miraculous—so you get premium heart power, without taking a second mortgage on your house. Plus, it's working to keep you healthy.

Every member of the "*Power 4*" helps to keep your ticker a heart of steel, but I want to show you how one in particular shines through as a personal hero of mine...

The Unbelievable link between curry and cholesterol

Honestly, I would never subject anyone to curry. I'm more of a steak and eggs man myself, but one ingredient found in the fragrant dish performs a feat I've never seen before.

There is a substance found in the Indian spice, turmeric, that could cause even me to have a culinary change of heart... It's called

curcumin and talk about smart—this one substance knows more about cholesterol than most
doctors I've run into.

While the research is preliminary, it appears that curcumin single-handedly promotes
healthy cholesterol and helps to keep your triglyceride levels healthy as an added bonus.
Take a look...

- In a 2011 human trial, 24 healthy volunteers took curcumin or the "miraculous"
  antioxidant vitamin E for just a week. And
  the curcumin group saw the biggest improvement in their cholesterol AND triglyceride
  levels—even more than the vitamin E group!

- It's been shown to increase the activity
  of an enzyme that breaks down cholesterol
  in vitro.

- It has *even* been shown to help support
  the heart in mice.

You see, in my opinion these two secrets
provide more heart support than the dozens and
dozens of "cardiovascular miracles" that have
been touted over the years.

While the studies are preliminary and mostly
in animals—you should not have to wait to have
these heart heroes working overtime for you.
Inflammation...blood pressure...cholesterol...
these two secrets could help push heart concerns out of you mind.

Individually, they pack enough heart health

support to keep you feeling strong and confident in your ticker... but I'm bringing them both together for the greatest heart health I've ever seen.

And speaking of...

Aside from you heart—nothing puts the "Father Time" fear in people more than losing your smarts. But when it comes to cutting-edge brain support—Ultra Vital Gold is years ahead of the competition.

How so? The answer is downright insulting...

Many memory protectors never even reach your brain.

As if charging too much for bloated, puffed up formulas wasn't bad enough... there are some "premium ingredients" that are just plain *super duds*.

I'll show you how the "Ultra Vital Gold difference" has your brain on track to keeping...

- Your memory popping, snapping and recalling memories with precision...

- Rock solid short-term memory—forget having to search for your keys, glasses and checkbook... and

- Cutting-edge protection that can have you feeling confident you're doing all you can to keep your brain firing on all cylinders...

The first step—and surprisingly, the step most other protectors fail to meet, is to get the goods right to where your brain will use them!

Your brain is your most important organ and as such—it's on more lock down than Fort Knox and the Oval Office combined. It's called the blood-brain barrier and it's a very tight weave of microscopic cells around the capillaries leading into your brain. Essentially, it's a concrete wall sandwiched between two steel doors designed to keep the bad guys out.

But this can be a problem for natural brain supporters because they can't make it through to begin with. Let me rephrase that... *some* natural brain supporters can't break through to the other side and give your brain the ultimate protection.

What's the secret code to get past the blood-brain barrier? It's tricky, but a select few can get through to provide the remarkable support to your brain power—and Ultra Vital Gold has the best. The Alpha Antioxidant is a very unique antioxidant (I told you the "Power 4" were multi-talented).

You see, antioxidants are either *water-soluble* or *fat-soluble* with each one able to travel to different areas of the body to hunt down free radicals.

But yet another "wow" factor with the Alpha Antioxidant is that it's both water-soluble and fat-soluble. That means it can pretty much go wherever it pleases—including past the blood brain barrier!

And once inside—the support it can deliver to your brain is huge. Once it's past the blood-brain barrier, it makes quick work of free radicals it comes across.

In one animal study, it lowered oxidative stress markers. And in yet another study where mice were given doses of astaxanthin equal to 10 mg for humans, it even supported memory health.

But, the fact that this is one of the few substances that can cross the "Red Alert" security system of your brain means it has INCREDIBLE potential in the research of memory support and cognitive health. Scientists are currently chomping at the bit to show the world its true potential. That's what convinced me we needed 4 mg of astaxanthin in each serving of Ultra Vital Gold!

You can start pumping the ultimate brain protection *deep into your brain* right now (While the other researchers of the world are just getting started), with my breakthrough formula.

And there's even MORE brain boosting in every capsule of Ultra Vital Gold. In fact, this next one was tailor made for mega mind maintenance—with the original brain booster. Why do I say the *original*? Because this next mind miracle plays a crucial role in the development of your brain.

DHA and EPA fatty acids are not only crucial in building your brain—but also keeping it strong, healthy and firing on all cylinders for your entire life.

Just take a look at these facts...

- DHA is a crucial element of the most abundant fatty acid in the human brain which makes up 50-60 percent of the brain's weight

- Breast-fed infants have been shown to have higher cognitive development—and what does mother's milk have a high concentration of? DHA.

- EPA AND DHA are able to lower triglycerides, which not only helps support the heart, but are also associated with better cognitive health

Sorry, but it's a no brainer to have DHA and EPA in any formula claiming to have benefits for your brain power. And these fatty acids are absolutely ESSENTIAL if you want to do all you can to support your brain from the inside-out.

With the "*Power 4*" keeping your heart and brain support in check—they're moving on to...

Bionic vision into your 70's, 80's and beyond

Just like your brain and heart, the "*Power 4*" found in Ultra Vital Gold rockets premium support right to where your eyes need it most. Now, the research has been performed in animal studies, but so far the results have shown this marvel ingredient's amazing potential... It supports vision health and conquers oxidative stress to help keep bionic vision. These three keys are the kind of protection that could equal healthy, strong, vibrant vision support for as long as you can imagine. It all starts with the final member of the Power 4 you have yet to meet, but I'm sure you've heard of...

The "comeback kid" of vitamins rushes revolutionary support to your eyes

Vitamin D has come a long way.

When I was growing up and would ask my mother why she made me drink so much milk, she would instantly reply, "the vitamin D builds strong bones."

That was more or less all science knew about it. But now, **what can't this vitamin powerhouse do?**

Heart health... your immune system... blood pressure... This vitamin seems to touch on just about every facet of your body's health—which makes it a perfect member of the Power 4. But when it comes to crystal clear vision, *vitamin D* kicks into high gear to keep vision sharp.

And just think...your heart, your brain, your eyes, and more—all protected by Ultra Vital Gold's *"Power 4"*.

Every second of every day these four medical marvels are diligently keeping watch over your body...

Much more than just an eye guardian—Vitamin D already has promising research results when it comes to... thyroid... skin... muscle strength... bone health... blood sugar support... even mood. And more studies are currently in the works with big results expected on the horizon.

Much more than just a heart hero—The Alpha Antioxidant has been put on the fast track in many research facilities because in just a short amount of time, it is creating waves in so many aspects of aging research. The preliminary animal and *in vitro* evidence shows the Alpha Antioxidant may help fight oxidative stress... promote a healthy inflammatory response... support immune system health... skin health... liver health and even athletic performance.

Much more than a brain booster—So now you know your brain and eyes heavily rely on DHA and EPA to stay packed with youth power, but that's just the start.

Joint health... weight control... healthy blood pressure... and endurance could all be supported with a healthy dose of DHA and EPA.

Even more than a heart helper—having just picked up steam here in the States, the Indian secret to longevity is fresh on the minds of America's greatest scientists since preliminary evidence is showing it's amazing potential. Joint concerns... cholesterol... healthy inflammation levels... detoxification... and supporting a healthy immune system all could be in this Indian sensation's sights! You can let it go to work for you today!

By my count... that's over 17 health concerns—and the Power 4 in Ultra Vital Gold takes them all to task!

I know it can be hard to believe that just *four ingredients* could do SO much to support your health, but now you've seen the evidence for yourself.

If you want to feel confident you will keep...

- **Living life *on your feet, out and about*, and ON THE GO**—instead of feeling like the sofa is your best friend...

- **Spending your days laughing, *loving* and listing off your favorite memories**—instead of sometimes struggling to recall minute details and facts...

- **Making the most of your *70's, 80's, 90's and more*** with hobbies, trips and the activities you love—instead of wishing you had the energy to get up and go...

Then you need the "*Power 4*" in every capsule of Ultra Vital Gold! (Go to page 410 for ordering information.)

Chapter 51:

Can This Anti-Aging Formula *Really* Help You Live 20 Percent Longer?

It sounds like hype—a magic potion that offers the possibility of living 20 percent longer.

And not just longer... better, too.

Your friends will see it on the outside. You'll feel it on the inside, energetic exuberance. You'll *know* it, because your mind will be sharper than ever... even if some memory loss has started kicking in.

Believe me, I know it sounds far-fetched, even impossible.

But HSI panelist Jon Barron has created just that: a true anti-aging formula that works to do all of those things... by rejuvenating every cell in your body.

Conquer these, and you conquer aging

There are so many things that make our bodies age, from stress to oxidation to hormone changes. But to really reverse the signs of aging, and maybe even extend life itself, there are two critical factors that until very recently scientists believed were completely irreversible.

The **Hayflick Limit** sets the life span of a cell. Basically, a cell can only divide so many times before it dies off. How many times depends on the type of cell—it's different for each type we have. But by the time we hit mid-life, far more than half of those divisions are used up. And when cells get very close to their end (but not at the end), they stop dividing—a state called senescence, the final step before cell death.

But some very exciting research tells us that the Hayflick Limit is no longer a cell death sentence... and cell aging can be reversed. But then there's still another big problem to deal with.

Glycation of proteins, also known as **cross-linking**, happens when sugars react with proteins. And since proteins are so crucial to every function in your body, anything that makes them deteriorate will have a gigantic impact on your activity and appearance. According to HSI Panelist Jon Barron, "Glycation is a major factor in the aging process—and it's particularly devastating to diabetics."

Scientists used to believe that damage was irreversible. And now we know—it's not.

Can one compound really reverse aging and extend life?

Let's get right into this.

The compound is L-carnosine (an amino acid combination), and the life extension research is nothing short of astonishing. It performs truly amazing magic at the cellular level.

- Reverses cell senescence, completing disregarding the Hayflick Limit

- Eliminates existing protein glycation and prevents more from ever taking place

- Reduces age-related telomere shortening and extends cell life span

- Stimulates stem cell production

How does that translate into whole-body benefits?

Groundbreaking research found that carnosine extended the lives of lab mice. And not only did the mice live much longer, they also lived "younger," with glossier coats and juvenile behaviors.[1,2]

A more recent study[3], this one using fruit flies—which, by the way, tell us a lot about aging because of their notoriously short life spans—found that their lives were extended by up to 20 percent when carnosine was added to their food.

Those studies came on the heels of *in vitro* studies, which broke scientifically shocking ground. When carnosine was added to old senescent cells in the lab, the cells got younger and began dividing again...extending cell life by up to 300 percent.

So it appears that carnosine can help you live longer and younger... and without fear of losing yourself.

What it does for your brain is truly miraculous

It's the scariest part of aging, what can happen to your brain. Alzheimer's disease and Parkinson's disease take a toll on you and the people you love. And there's virtually nothing mainstream medicine or Big Pharma can do about it.

But L-carnosine can do a lot, especially in combination with the other key ingredients in Jon Barron's Ever Young formula. Together with acetyl-L-carnitine (ALC) and DMAE, this anti-aging formula doesn't just turn back the clock on your appearance. These ingredients truly fight the causes of aging and deterioration, especially in your brain.

For one thing, carnosine has been shown to limit, even completely prevent, the brain damage caused by beta amyloid—a key factor in Alzheimer's disease.[4]

On top of that, ALC brings a very long list of brain benefits to the formula, thanks to its ability to cross the blood-brain barrier.

- Preserves and protects brain cells

- Improves alertness and cognition in

Alzheimer's patients[5].

- Improves dopamine processing, and seems to help minimize Parkinson's disease symptoms

- Improves long and short term memory

- Slows down brain aging

DMAE (dimethylaminoethanol) adds different support for your brain, primarily in its role as the precursor of a critical brain chemical called acetylcholine. A lot of research has been done on DMAE and its link to increased brain power. Just some of the things it can do...

- Improve concentration and attention span

- Increase intelligence

- Boost memory

- Put you in a better mood

- Make it easier to fall asleep, and help you sleep more soundly

And DMAE also brings something very rare to the formula.

The truly unique function of DMAE

Age spots on your skin are easy to see. But it's those brown age spots on your organs— known as lipofuscin—that you need to worry about.

Lipofuscin is basically the cellular waste left by free radical damage. And if you can see those spots on your skin, it's a sign they're inside, too—on your liver, heart, and even your brain.

Enter DMAE, which dissolves lipofuscin, both inside and out. It works by flushing accumulated lipofuscin out of your entire body, from the back of your hand and from your brain cells.

Take Ever Young to turn back the clock both inside and out

Finally, an anti-aging formula that works to rejuvenate your very cells, keeping you young and vital inside and out.

The manufacturer recommends taking one or two capsules of Ever Young three times a day. To avoid potential minor side effects (like mild headache), start with a lower dose and work your way up to the full daily dose.

And just so you know, Ever Young™ may have a strong vinegar-like smell from the acetyl complex in the Acetyl-L-Carnitine. Keeping it in the refrigerator can lessen that.

You can find ordering information for Ever Young in your Wellness Directory on page 409.

Chapter 52:

Junk Science Gone Wild: Are Your Supplements Driving You Blind?

Now here is some junk science I can really love to hate. It's so corny, so absurd, so un-scientific, so fecalithic that we can only laugh hysterically and ask these intellectual/scientific twerps for more.

"Many herbal remedies and nutritional supplements can damage the eyes, including some alternative therapies that are used by people trying to correct eye problems... According to a review of reported cases and medical literature, commonly used supplements including chamomile, ginkgo biloba, licorice, vitamin A and echinacea can cause a myriad of eye problems," reports *Reuters Health*. Study author Dr. Frederick Fraunfelder explained to *Reuters* that "supplements become dangerous to the eyes when people take them in large doses." The primary "dangers" Fraunfelder cited are retinal bleeding, conjunctivitis, and temporary vision loss—all from, he claims, vitamins, and herbs.

"Tell your physician what you take, as these products interact with other drugs," Fraunfelder advises. "Recognize even herbal products and nutritional supplements have adverse reactions." To hide his bias, Frederick should say "could have" adverse reactions, don't you think?

Blaming supplements for retinal bleeding is a pretty bold move, considering every time you take an aspirin or a dose of Coumadin prescribed by a doctor—not an overdose but a recommended dose—you bleed a little in your gut, your brain, your bladder, or possibly your eye.

"People who choose to take supplements that can damage eyes should schedule an eye exam before beginning the treatment, then visit an eye doctor every year to monitor their eyes," he told *Reuters Health*. Notice he isn't recommending that you get this exam before taking the doctor's known hemorrhage-inducing drugs but only if you are anticipating taking an herbal or other nutrient that, when taken in the recommended dosage, causes few if any side effects. How many times has a doctor recommended that you take an annual eye exam if you are taking aspirin daily?

Yes, you should tell your doctor what you are taking so that (once he looks it up) he can advise you as to whether there is a conflict between drugs he knows (or should know) cause bleeding and the nutrients you are taking. But most people are intimidated by doctors and don't want to be ridiculed or chastised for taking the natural approach, so they remain silent.

The difference between correlation, causation, and conjecture

The other specific instances of eye damage Fraunfelder points out are just as ridiculous as the bleeding claim—maybe more so.

He indicts canthaxanthine for causing negative changes in the retina, including crystal deposits. I don't know if Fraunfelder is confusing correlation with causation or not, but, first of all, canthaxanthine is a natural pigment in carrots used most commonly for sunless tanning. But in order for it to cause any changes in the body, you have to eat enormous amounts of it. And even then, the worst that can really happen is you'll turn orange. Besides, anyone who uses anything like this to induce an orangish suntan is either naïve or stupid—or excessively vain.

Then *Reuters Health* reports: "The researcher uncovered seven cases in which people rinsed their eyes with chamomile tea to treat styes and irritation, and instead developed severe conjunctivitis." This is just silly and illustrates how "science" and their handmaiden, the press, mislead people into seeing problems that are trivial or essentially nonexistent. A stye is a little pimple on the lower lid of the eye. It is not a threat to the eye or to the patient in any way. The chamomile tea is worthless (in my opinion) but probably harmless. The best way to treat a stye is with a hot compress—just close your eye and apply hot compresses to it every 20 minutes. If it doesn't seem to be improving after 24 hours, go to an ophthalmologist, who will prick it with a needle, which will greatly shorten the healing time—especially if you continue using the hot compresses. When the stye ruptures, the pus inside will flow over into the eyeball. Gross, yes, but not to worry; the hot compresses will heal it, and the doctor will usually prescribe eye drops containing an antibiotic and cortisone that will probably shorten the healing time even more. That's all there is to it.

Then there's echinacea, which, according to the article, "is widely touted as useful for treating the common cold and flu, but Fraunfelder found several cases in which users developed irritation and conjunctivitis after using it topically." How does Fraunfelder know the "irritation and conjunctivitis" were caused by the echinacea? Were the patients <u>rubbing it into their eyes</u> to treat a cold? When people use products—natural or not—in ways outside their intended purpose, you can hardly blame the product for causing the problem—not that it necessarily did in this case.

"The researcher also discovered five cases of temporary vision loss apparently caused by licorice consumption." Oo-oo-wee! Better stay away from that licorice. Well, not necessarily.

Licorice (in its all-natural form, not Twizzlers) has been used for hundreds of years and has millions of proponents worldwide. What Fraunfelder does not say, and probably doesn't know, is that the <u>deglycerinated</u> form of licorice is quite safe. It may cause a temporary rise in blood pressure in some patients, but I have never heard of glycerin causing a "temporary vision loss," and I suggest that the researchers prove their case. Reporting that it "apparently caused" vision loss is not science, it's conjecture.

The report also indicts niacin, ginkgo biloba, and vitamin A ("a particularly big threat") as vision killers. None of these is a threat to your health in any way if taken in acceptable doses.

Actions to take:

(1) As with powerful and dangerous pharmaceuticals, don't take excessive doses of nutrients or anything else, including water, exercise, TV, and sex.

(2) Ask your pharmacist to look up possible interactions between your prescription drugs and the nutrients that you are taking.

P.S. Anticipating a letter to the editor: "What does 'fecalithic' mean?" Answer: a "fecalith" is a teeny-tiny calcified doo-doo ball found in the colon. And that's about the level of importance of this innuendo-laden and sophomoric report.

Chapter 53:

I'M STILL STANDING!
Leading Cause of Falls in Seniors
Isn't Age—It's Drugs
Your Guide to Common Pitfalls and How
to Avoid Them

Hit a certain age, and your doctor will just stop listening. Sure, he'll make all the usual sympathetic noises—but really, he's waiting for you to shut up so he can deliver his pre-rehearsed answer:

You're just getting older.

Of course, Father Time can do a number on anyone—but some of the leading medical problems facing seniors today aren't a product of age.

Just look at falls. Every year, a third of all seniors take a tumble, leading to 2 million hospitalizations and 20,000 deaths—but age alone isn't what's making old folks stumble around like drunks on a Friday night.

It's drugs—drugs that can leave you woozy, wobbly, dizzy, and unsteady.

Take enough meds, and a fall is practically inevitable—and even if you survive, you could face shattered bones, crippling pain, lifelong disability, a loss of independence, and a downward spiral that could ultimately end in the grave.

I've been tracking the research on falls for years now, and I've identified the three Prime Suspects responsible for the lion's share of all this pain and misery.

These drugs are so common that you or someone you love is almost certainly on at least one of them. Maybe even all three.

But here's your chance to get off them for good—because I'm not just naming names today. I'm also going to give you the BETTER and SAFER options that can accomplish everything those drugs can... but with none of the risk.

PRIME SUSPECT #1: PAINKILLERS

Narcotic painkillers can leave you so loopy that even if you do fall, you might not care. You'll just lie on the floor until the drug wears off—and when you come to, you literally won't know what hit you.

But instead of moving to get seniors off these drugs, many docs are putting more on them. Back in 2001, just 8 percent of osteoarthritis patients were on opioid painkillers. By 2005, 20 percent were on these meds. And in 2009, a full **40 percent** of osteoarthritis patients were stoned on opioid painkillers.

Want to know what else happened in that time? The number of falls and fractures among those same patients tripled, from less than 1 percent in 2001 to 4 percent in 2009.

THE FALL-FREE SOLUTION: Mainstream researchers claim the best way to get seniors off opioid painkillers is by shifting them onto stomach-wrecking anti-inflammatory meds such as ibuprofen instead.

Then, to undo some of the stomach damage, they want to give everyone a lifetime supply of proton pump inhibitors—drugs that could suck the calcium right out of your bones, making it **_more likely_** they'll snap even if you don't fall.

You just can't make this stuff up!

So forget ibuprofen, and pass on the opioids. Curcumin, a natural anti-inflammatory compound, is proven to bring just as much pain relief as drugs in osteoarthritis patients, and you can bet it works for other forms of pain as well.

You can also try other natural anti-inflammatories such as fish oil. But more importantly, work with a doc who can actually find the cause of your pain and correct it instead of one who just wants to give you some pills and send you on your way.

To find the name of a doc near you I recommend the American College for Advancement in Medicine: Online at ACAM.org or call 1-800-532-3688.

PRIME SUSPECT #2: MOOD MEDS

Psychiatric drugs have become some of the

nation's best-selling meds—especially antide-pressants, antipsychotics, and benzodiazepines and seniors are getting more than their share of those prescriptions.

In many cases—especially those antipsychot-ics—seniors are given the drugs off-label, for conditions where the drugs aren't even proven to work.

But while the drugs might do nothing for the condition itself, they can still pack plenty of side effects, including **DOUBLE** the risk of falling, according to one recent study. Not just once or twice, mind you. That would be bad enough—but the study finds these drugs double your risk of falling ***three or more times*** over the course of a single year.

You know the score on that. Any fall can be your last. But three or more? That's a risk you shouldn't take—and it's a risk you don't have to take, because you've got better options.

THE FALL-FREE SOLUTION: First, we need to end the nonsensical idea that every single emo-tion needs to be chemically controlled.

Sometimes, the best thing to do with de-pression and anxiety is the let them run their course. It's part of the human experience, and time itself will often heal these wounds. If that doesn't do the trick, a weekend in a place with the word "beach" in the name might be just what the doctor ordered.

And if you need a little more help getting

over the hump, try natural brain-supporting supplements such as fish oil and acetyl L-carnitine. A little St. John's wort or valerian can also help, although more serious cases may call for hormone supplementation under the care of a naturopathic physician.

PRIME SUSPECT #3: SLEEP DRUGS

Sleep meds such as Ambien could make you so loopy that the FDA recently admitted you might be unfit to drive not just right after taking them (of course) but as late as ***THE NEXT MORNING.***

And if that's how sleep drugs impair your driving abilities up to 8 hours later, just imagine what they do to your walking abilities when you get up for a late-night potty run.

A Mayo Clinic study of hospitalized seniors found that patients taking Ambien had quadruple the risk of falls, and a Harvard study of nursing home patients found Ambien and similar sleep meds increased the risk of hip fractures by 66 percent in the first 30 days, almost certainly due to that fall risk.

You don't have to be in a care facility to face this hazard. All you need is a sleep med and the need to walk somewhere in the night—even if it's just a few steps to the bathroom door.

THE FALL-FREE SOLUTION: Sleep problems can often be corrected with hormone supplementation. Over-the-counter melatonin will work for many, but others may require supplementation with HGH under the care of an experienced naturopath.

Those aren't all the drugs that can increase your fall risk. Just the Big Three—but others can do the job just as efficiently, including seizure meds, sedatives (or any drug with a sedative side effect), allergy and cold meds, antihistamines, cough remedies, and more.

And in many cases it's not a single drug. Most seniors are given enough meds to sedate a moose—and the more you take, the more unsteady you'll be.

Minimize those meds, and you'll minimize your risk. But don't stop there. There are other easy actions you can take right now to make sure every step is steady, starting with a step out your front door and into the sunlight.

That's where you'll get vitamin D, the hormone proven to reduce the risk of falls by 22 percent—and since the sunshine vitamin is also known to strengthen bone and muscle, you'll be less likely to get hurt if you do take a spill.

Finally, invite your kids and grandkids over for a redecorating party. It's as good an excuse as any for that long-overdue family gathering. They can check the railing on the staircase, install grab bars in the bathroom and shower, fix that broken step on the porch, and help look around for other potential fall hazards like area rugs.

No one likes to admit that being older means being a little more careful, but there's no shame in making a few basic safety changes. The real shame would be in what happens if you don't.

Chapter 54:

KILLING YOU SOFTLY
Death and Dementia in the Drugs You Take Every Day!

It's death where you least expect it: Right in your own medicine chest, as the common drugs taken by millions of seniors each day may damage the brain, cause dementia or delirium, and even **_kill_** you.

You won't find this risk listed on the label, and don't expect your doctor to warn you about it. Heck, he might not even be aware of it.

That's what you have me for—so let me tell you what he won't about a class of drugs called anticholinergics.

The name might not be all that familiar. But the drugs themselves are—because you've almost certainly taken them at some point in your life.

You may even be on them right now, because anticholinergics include some of the most commonly used meds on the planet: cold medications, painkillers, antidepressants, blood thinners, allergy and asthma drugs, antihistamines, and more.

Different drugs. Different illnesses. Different names. Some are available by prescription. Others, right over the counter.

But anticholinergic drugs all have one thing in common: They block acetylcholine, a key chemical in the brain.

It's bad enough to screw with your acetylcholine levels by taking even one of these drugs. But take two, three, four, or more—as many seniors do—and it's a small wonder you can even think straight.

It doesn't take long for the brain damage to sink in, either. Seniors who take three anticholinergics or more could have TRIPLE the risk of mild cognitive impairment in just 90 days, according to one study.

Taking even two drugs for 60 days can DOUBLE your risk.

That's the fast track to a slow mind, my friend—and the risks don't get any better from there. Another study showed that taking even a single anticholinergic med for six years could increase your overall risk of this brain-robbing condition by 46 percent.

And the sky's the limit after that—because the more anticholinergic drugs you take, the higher your risk of cognitive decline.

These aren't risks that have popped up in a

study or two here and there. One review found a link between anticholinergic meds and either dementia, cognitive impairment, or delirium *in 25 out of 27 studies*.

But you've got to admit, even a slower brain is better than one that's flatlined—and that's the other, BIGGER risk here, because these drugs may not only be associated with cognitive decline, dementia, and delirium.

No, there's one other D—the "big" D:

DEATH

Regular use of these drugs upped the odds of death by 68 percent for heavy users, according to the recent study in *The Journal of the American Geriatrics Society*.

The more you take, the higher your risk—with each anticholinergic "point" potentially upping your odds of death by 26 percent, and just taking one known anticholinergic could up your risk for cognitive impairment by 46 percent.

The "point" system is how you can calculate your overall anticholinergic burden. Since some drugs are known to be anticolinergic and some are just suspected, the ones that have more powerful anticholinergic effects than others get more points.

At the "low" end are one-point drugs that are possible anticholinergics such as Valium, Xanax, and the blood thinner warfarin. At the high end, you'll find three-point drugs such as Benadryl, Dimetapp, and common cough meds as well as everything from the antipsychotic drug Seroquel to the bladder control med Ditropan.

The list includes so many meds that 20 percent of America's seniors are on at least one of them at any given time. That's 7 million Americans taking one or more potentially brain-slowing, life-robbing drugs every day—and you or your loved ones could be among them.

So right now, it's absolutely urgent that you take these three simple steps to protect yourself and your loved ones from dementia, delirium, and an early grave:

- **Learn** which drugs are anticholinergic and which are not. This isn't as easy as it sounds, because there are about a billion of them—or more than I can list here, anyway. Google "anticholinergic burden" to find some lists. Since the lists vary, read several of them. Better yet, call your doctor pronto and make him tell you. That's why you pay him, right?

- **Watch** for over-the-counter meds, because easy availability doesn't mean safe. Some of the worst-of-the-worst anticholinergic drugs... one's that are high on the "point" system... are available without a prescription, including the Benadryl and Dimetapp I just mentioned.

- **Find** alternatives. In most cases, you don't even need those anticholinergic drugs in the first place. The blood thinner warfarin, for example, can often be swapped with cod liver oil—and instead of slowing your brain, cod liver oil can actually protect it.

But whatever you do, don't fly solo here. Any time you start, stop or swap a drug, you need to do it with the help of a doctor—and these meds are no exception, since many of them pack the extra punch of withdrawal symptoms.

I recommend working with an experienced member of the American College for Advancement in Medicine. Go online to ACAM.org or call 1-800-532-3688 to find the name of a doc near you.

Chapter 55:

How to Survive Any Disaster

Sometimes, I can't tell if I'm reading the news or the plots of Hollywood disaster flicks.

We've got superstorms, supergerms, terror plots, and industrial accidents that can wipe entire towns off the map—and God only knows what kind of threats tomorrow will bring.

Sometimes, it seems like you need to be James Bond to survive one of these disasters. But I like your odds here—because you've got someone even craftier than Q in your corner.

You've got me.

So take a day this summer to skip the movies and engage in something far more important. Prepare yourself and your family for a disaster, using my...

FOUR STEPS TO SURVIVAL

STEP ONE: Make sure your home is ready for a shelter-in-place if necessary. Stock up on extra food such as emergency rations or MREs, gallons of water, battery-powered radios (and batteries), flashlights, a first-aid kit, generator, fuel, and more. If you've got a pet, make sure you've got supplies for your critter, too.

I know this isn't politically correct, but you also want a firearm and the ability to use it. If things really go south, you don't want to be without a weapon.

Keep all your supplies in the attic, if you have one, and not the basement if you live in an area prone to flooding. And if flood is a threat, make sure your attic has an axe so you can hack your way out if necessary as well as a self-inflating raft.

STEP TWO: If you're near any kind of ominous plant—a nuclear facility, chemicals plant, fertilizer factory, etc.—have three or four routes out of town memorized, and practice your evacuation plan. You want to be able to get out the door and on the road in 10 minutes or less—and clear out of town without using any major highways.

Those will clog long before the warning sirens sound.

STEP THREE: Have plenty of cash on hand. If you need to travel during a disaster, you'll need plenty of it—and you won't have time to stop at an ATM. Even if they're working, you can bet the lines will be around the block.

If you're smart, you'll also have some precious metals such as gold. If things REALLY hit the fan, your paper currency will be even more worthless than it is today.

A fireproof safe isn't a bad idea for storing this stuff.

STEP FOUR: Make sure your family has a place to meet if disaster strikes while you're out and you can't reach your home. Ideally, choose a friend or relative's house, away from any well-known landmarks and in the opposite direction of potential threats such as raging rivers, nuclear plants, and Washington D.C.

Don't count on your phone to keep in touch. If there's a disaster, your smart phone will almost certainly go dumb.

And if anyone is less dependable than Ma Bell, it's Uncle Sam. As Katrina taught us too well, he'll leave you up a creek without a paddle (or even a raft), and then throw you a concrete block for a lifeline.

So don't count on either of them for help.

As always, the only one you can truly depend on (besides me) is yourself—and your own ability to prepare.

Chapter 56:

HOW TO SURVIVE OBAMACARE:
Your Guide to the Ugly Future
of Medicine

Seen the lines at the doctor's office lately?

Those lines aren't being caused by the flu. They're being caused by something worse—a disease that's laid waste to entire nations. It's a festering sickness called socialism.

ObamaCare hasn't even fully kicked in yet, but doctors are already feeling the strain of growing patient enrollments and not enough time to see them all. It's so bad that many physicians are no longer accepting new patients.

We're not just short by a few doctors here and there. We're short by thousands, and in the fields you and your family depend on most—including primary care, internal medicine, geriatrics, and pediatrics.

It's so bad that within two years, this "doctor deficit" is going to hit 62,900—and by 2025, we'll be short by 100,000 doctors, according to the latest estimates from the Association of

American Medical Colleges.

And that's WITHOUT considering the effects of ObamaCare. Once this nation-wrecking socialist scheme fully kicks in and 30 million new patients get "free" access to YOUR doctor ("free" for them, that is, because YOU'RE paying for it) the doctor deficit is expected to hit 140,000.

Isn't that outrageous? People forced to pay into the system won't be able to get anywhere near their own doctors... while moochers with "free" ObamaCare will have complete access whenever they need it.

Of course, the Obama Administration says it wouldn't dream of adding 30 million new patients to the rolls without funding education for more doctors—so they're working hard to add thousands of new physicians.

Three thousand, to be exact, spread out over a decade. You don't need a calculator to know that'll leave us 137,000 doctors short—and even that could be a wildly optimistic number, because a third of today's doctors are 55 years old or older, according to a recent report in the **New York Times**.

They're approaching retirement age—and you can bet that many of them will start hanging up their stethoscopes early once they see the growing lines outside their door and shrinking reimbursements in their paychecks.

Don't wait for the shortage to grow before

you take action. Protect yourself and your family with these three steps:

1) If you don't have a primary care doctor yet, find one **fast**. Already I'm hearing from readers across the country that it's almost impossible to find a doctor who's accepting new patients. That's going to get even harder, not easier, so find yours now.

2) Once you do have a doctor, get to know him and get on his good side so he'll be there for you when you need him.

3) Get to know the front office staff and get on their good side, too—especially the one who keeps the appointment book. Don't be afraid to send flowers and boxes of candy. You can bet someone else will—and he'll get an appointment anytime he needs one.

But there's another option here—and that's to skip the lines and see a doctor who doesn't have them in the first place. Socialism may be spreading like a disease throughout medicine, but there's one branch that's practically immune—and that's NATURAL medicine.

You see, ObamaCare is being run through insurance companies, and since many insurers actually consider natural medicine to be a form of fraud, most of them won't even deal with naturopaths.

That means you'll have to pay a little more

out of pocket, of course. But in return, you'll get appointments when you need them and real solutions instead of a few quick squiggles on a prescription pad. In short, you'll get a doctor who actually has time for you.

Imagine that! Now, stop imagining and contact the American College for Advancement in Medicine to find the name of a doctor near you. Visit them online at acam.org or call 1-800-532-3688.

Wellness Directory

AquaFlora High Potency 9, KingBio. Tel: (888) 827-6414; www.kingbio.com. AquaFlora High Potency 9 costs US$32.99, and the three support formulas (AquaFlora Probiotic, AquaFlora Enzyme, AquaFlora Heavy Metal Detox) each cost US$25.99.

AvéULTRA™, The Harmony Company. Tel: (800)422-5518; www.theharmonycompany.com.

Bacopa, Himalaya Pure Herbs. Tel: (855)665-8449; www.himalayausa.com. Bacopa costs US$18.95 for a bottle of 60 caplets. Product only available in the U.S.

Ever Young, Baseline Nutritionals. Tel: (800)440-3120; www.baselinenutritionals.com. Ever Young costs $89.95 for a 180-count bottle. Please note: Phone lines are open only from 9:00 a.m. to 4:00 p.m. Pacific Standard Time, Monday to Friday.

GlucoComplete, Real Advantage Nutrients. Tel: (888)856-1491; www.realadvantagenutrients.com. Save 20 percent when you order by using code G655P803.

Graviola, Raintree Nutrition, Inc. www.rain-tree.com.

ImmPower™, The Harmony Company. Tel: (800)422-5518; www.theharmonycompany.com.

N-Tense, Raintree Nutrition, Inc. www.rain-tree.com.

ONCOblot® Test, ONCOblot Labs. Tel: (765)464-1583; www.oncoblotlabs.com. The ONCOblot® Test costs $850, and must be ordered by a physician. Your physician can order the kit using the above contact information. Or you can order through one of these physicians:

- Dr. Leigh Erin Connealy, MD, (949)680-1880
  www.centerfornewmedicine.com
- Dr. Claudia Hanau, ND, (765)464-1545
  www.hanauholistic.com
- Dr. Kimberly Wilson, NMD, (972)608-0100
  www.innovationswellness.com

Red Bee Propolis, NaturaNectar. Tel. (800)609-7794; www.NaturaNectar.com. Red Bee Propolis costs US$74.94 for a 60-day supply.

Ultimate Bionic Plus, Real Advantage Nutrients. Tel: (888)856-1491; www.realadvantagenutrients.com. Save 20 percent when you order by using code G655P804.

Ultimate PRO Support, Real Advantage Nutrients. Tel: (888)856-1491; www.realadvantagenutrients.com. Save 20 percent when you order by using code G655P809.

Ultimate Tendon Support, Real Advantage Nutrients. Tel: (888)856-1491; www.realadvantagenutrients.com. Save 20 percent when you order by using code G655P805.

Ultimate Vigor, Real Advantage Nutrients. Tel: (888)856-1491; www.realadvantagenutrients.com. Save 20 percent when you order by using code G655P806.

Ultra Turbo HG, Real Advantage Nutrients. Tel: (888)856-1491; www.realadvantagenutrients.com. Save 20 percent when you order by using code G655P807.

Ultra Vital Gold, Real Advantage Nutrients. Tel: (888)856-1491; www.realadvantagenutrients.com. Save 20 percent when you order by using code G655P808.

References

Chapter 1: When I First Hear About This, I Was Furious! The One Cancer
Test That Could Save Your Life...If Only You Knew About It

[1] Brandon Hostetler, et al. Cancer Site-Specific Isoforms of ENOX2
(tNOX), A Cancer-Specific Cell Surface Oxidase. Clinical Proteomics,
March 2009, Volume 5, Issue 1, pp 46-51.

Chapter 2: The Number One Treatment I'd Use for ANY Cancer Patient,
Even Advanced Stage Melanoma Patients Live Years Longer and Better
with This 'Miracle' Compound

[1] Demidov LV, et al., Adjuvant fermented wheat germ extract (Avemar)
nutraceutical improves survival of high-risk skin melanoma patients: a
randomized, pilot, phase II clinical study with a 7-year follow-up, Cancer
Biother Radiopharm. 2008 Aug;23(4):477-82.

[2] Jakab, F., et al., A medical nutriment study has supportive effect in oral
cancer. British Journal of Cancer (2003), 89:465-469.

[3] "Fermented wheat germ extract inhibits glycolysis/pentose cycle enzymes
and induces apoptosis throughpoly(ADP-ribose) polymerase activation in
Jurkat T-cell leukemia tumor cells." Journal of Biological Chemistry 2002;
277: 46,408-46,414.

[4] "Fermented wheat germ extract induces apoptosis and downregulation
of major complex class I proteins in tumor T and B cell lines." International Journal of Oncology 2002; 20: 563-570.

[5] Sukkar, S., et al., A multicentric prospective open trial on the quality of
life and oxidative stress in patients affected by advanced head and neck
cancer treated with new benzoquinone-rich product derived from fermented wheat germ (Avemar). Mediterr J Nutr Metab, 2008.

[6] "A medical nutrient has supportive value in the treatment of colorectal
cancer." British Journal of Cancer Aug 4; 89(3): 465-9.

[7] Ghoneum M., Et Al., Immunomodulatory and Anticancer Effects of
Active Hemicellulose Compound (Ahcc), Int. J. Immunotherapy X1(1)
23-28 (1995).

Chapter 3: Rare Brazilian Compound Takes on Free Radicals, Infections,
and Even the Most Deadly Cancer

[1] Awale S, Constituents of Brazilian red propolis and their preferential
cytotoxic activity against human pancreatic PANC-1 cancer cell line in

nutrient-deprived condition. Bioorg Med Chem. 2008 Jan 1;16(1):181-9. Epub 2007 Oct 5.

[2] Li F, et al., Cytotoxic constituents from Brazilian red propolis and their structure-activity relationship.Bioorg Med Chem. 2008 May 15;16(10):5434-40. Epub 2008 Apr 12.

[3] Franchi, GC Jr., et al. Comparison of effects of the ethanolic extracts of brazilian propolis on human leukemic cells as assesed with the MTT assay. Evid Based Complement Alternat Med. 2012; 2012:918-956.

[4] Dota KF, et al., Antifungal Activity of Brazilian Propolis Microparticles against Yeasts Isolated from Vulvovaginal Candidiasis.

Evid Based Complement Alternat Med. 2011;2011:201953. Epub 2011 Mar 9.

Chapter 18: Three Reasons You Don't Need "Regular" Prostate-Cancer Screening

"Variation of Serum Prostate-Specific Antigen Levels: An Evaluation of Year-to-Year Fluctuations," Journal of the American Medical Association 2003; 289(20): 2,695-2,700.

"Study Recommends 2nd Test Before a Prostate Biopsy," The New York Times, 5/29/03 (section A, page 17).

Chapter 21: Eat All the Fried Food You Want Without Feeling Guilty or Increasing Your Heart Attack Risk

"Fish Consumption and Stroke Risk in Elderly Individuals," Archives of Internal Medicine 2005; 165(2): 200-206.

"Fried Fish Raises Stroke Risk: Broiled or baked reduces it, study finds," HealthDayNews, 1/24/05.

Chapter 27: New Research Shows Age-Related Blindness Can Be Prevented—With Food

"Dietary fat and fish intake and age-related maculopathy," Archives of Ophthalmology 2000; 118(3): 401-404.

Chapter 35: Cut Your Diabetes Risk by 83 Percent by Choosing the Right Beverages

Sugar-sweetened soft drinks, obesity, and type 2 diabetes," JAMA 2004; 292(8): 978-979.

Chapter 37: The Nutrition Lesson 100 Years in the Making: Learn It Now and Stay Diabetes-Free for Good

"Increased consumption of refined carbohydrates and the epidemic of type 2 diabetes in the United States: an ecologic assessment," American Journal of Clinical Nutrition 2004; 79(5): 774-779.

"Study Blames Corn Syrup for Rise of Diabetes in US," Reuters Health News, 4/22/04.

Chapter 38: Could You Be the Next Victim of Syndrome X, or—Even Worse—Syndrome H?

"1/3 of Americans Have Pre-diabetes Syndrome: Report," Reuters Health news, 8/27/02.

"Findings and Recommendations from the American College of Endocrinology Conference on the Insulin Resistance Syndrome" American Association of Clinical Endocrinologists (press release), 8/26/02.

Chapter 42: Big Pharma Hopes You Never Find Out About This Ayurvedic Herb That Puts Alzheimer's Drugs to Shame

[1] Neuropsychopharmacology. 2002 Aug;27(2):279-81. Chronic effects of Brahmi (Bacopa monnieri) on human memory. Roodenrys S.

[2] J Altern Complement Med. 2010 Jul;16(7):753-9. doi: 10.1089/ acm.2009.0342. Does Bacopa monnieri improve memory performance in older persons? Results of a randomized, placebo-controlled, double-blind trial. Morgan A, Stevens J.

[3] Stough C, Phytother Res. 2008 Dec;22(12):1629-34. doi: 10.1002/ ptr.2537. Examining the nootropic effects of a special extract of Bacopa monniera on human cognitive functioning: 90 day double-blind placebo-controlled randomized trial.

[4] J Ayurveda Integr Med. 2012 Oct;3(4):223-5. doi: 10.4103/0975-9476.104448. Add-on effect of Brahmi in the management of schizophrenia. Sarkar S.

[5] Psychopharmacology (Berl). 2013 May;227(2):299-306. doi: 10.1007/ s00213-013-2978-z. Epub 2013 Jan 26. Brahmi for the better? New findings challenging cognition and anti-anxiety effects of Brahmi (Bacopa monniera) in healthy adults. Sathyanarayanan V.

[6] Evid Based Complement Alternat Med. 2012;2012:606424. doi: 10.1155/2012/606424. Epub 2012 Dec 18. Effects of 12-Week Bacopa monnieri Consumption on Attention, Cognitive Processing, Working

Memory, and Functions of Both Cholinergic and Monoaminergic Systems in Healthy Elderly Volunteers. Peth-Nui T.

[7] Fundam Clin Pharmacol. 2013 Feb;27(1):96-103. doi: 10.1111/fcp.12000. Epub 2012 Oct 3. Na(+) -K(+) -ATPase, a potent neuroprotective modulator against Alzheimer disease. Zhang LN.

[8] Neurochem Res. 2012 Sep;37(9):1928-37. doi: 10.1007/s11064-012-0811-4. Epub 2012 Jun 15. Neuroprotective effects of Bacopa monnieri in experimental model of dementia. Saini N.

[9] J Ethnopharmacol. 2010 Jan 8;127(1):26-31. doi: 10.1016/j.jep.2009.09.056. Epub 2009 Oct 4. Cognitive enhancement and neuroprotective effects of Bacopa monnieri in Alzheimer's disease model. Uabundit N.

Chapter 44: Have You Been a Guinea Pig for the Latest, "Greatest" Surgical Scams? Read This Before You Go Under the Knife!

"Common Knee Surgery Is Found to Be Worthless" Wall Street Journal online (www.wsj.com), 7/11/02.

"A Controlled Trial of Arthroscopic Surgery for Osteoarthritis of the Knee," New England Journal of Medicine 2002; 347(2): 81-88.

Chapter 48: Can This Anti-Aging Formula Really Help You Live 20 Percent Longer?

[1] Shao L, Li QH, Tan Z., L-carnosine reduces telomere damage and shortening rate in cultured normal fibroblasts., Biochem Biophys Res Commun. 2004 Nov 12;324(2):931-6.

[2] Corona C, Effects of dietary supplementation of carnosine on mitochondrial dysfunction, amyloid pathology, and cognitive deficits in 3xTg-AD mice. PLoS One. 2011 Mar 15;6(3):e17971. doi: 10.1371/journal.pone.0017971.

[3] Boldyrev AA, Gallant SC, Sukhich GT. Carnosine, the protective, anti-aging peptide. Biosci Rep. 1999 Dec;19(6):581-7.

[4] Gallant S, Semyonova M, Yuneva M. Carnosine as a potential anti-senescence drug. Biochemistry (Mosc). 2000 Jul;65(7):866-8.

[5] Stvolinsky S, Antipin M, Meguro K, Sato T, Abe H, Boldyrev A. Effect of carnosine and its Trolox-modified derivatives on lifespan of Drosophila melanogaster. Rejuvenation Res. 2010 Aug;13(4):453-7.

[6] Wang AM, Use of carnosine as a natural anti-senescence drug for human beings.Biochemistry (Mosc). 2000 Jul;65(7):869-71.

[7] De Jesus Moreno, Cognitive improvement in mild to moderate Alzheimer's dementia after treatment with the acetylcholine precursor choline alfoscerate: a multicenter, double-blind, randomized, placebo-controlled trial. Clin Ther. 2003 Jan;25(1):178-93.

Chapter 49: Junk Science Gone Wild: Are Your Supplements Driving You Blind?

"Ocular side effects from herbal medicines and nutritional supplements," American Journal of Ophthalmology 2004; 138(4): 639-647.

"Some supplements can damage eyes," Reuters Health News (www.reuters.com), 10/21/04.